The Pox Doctor's Clerk

Walter Cockshaw

The Pox Doctor's Clerk

by

Walter Cockshaw

New Millennium
292 Kennington Road, London SE11 4LD

British Library Cataloguing in Publication Data.
A catalogue record for this book is available from the British Library.

Printed by Watkiss Studios Ltd. Biggleswade, Bedfordshire.
Issued by New Millennium*
ISBN 1 85845 176 0
*An imprint of The Professional Authors' & Publishers' Association

Dedicated to the staff of the Accident and Emergency Department at the Leicester Royal Infirmary and to my friends Iris, Jack, Barbara, Mike and Joy.

Contents

Author's Notes

Certain associations we experience during our lifetime, such as love and friendship, are always engraved in our memories, and other bonds we forge are also retained. It is for this reason I have recorded the incidents linked together in this book, which covers a period of over twenty years of voluntary work in the Accident and Emergency Department of a busy hospital in Central England.

All the incidents are true, but for obvious reasons the names of all the characters mentioned in these pages have been changed. The whole spectrum of human behaviour is covered and for some, the unwanted and the unloved, who are no longer with us, these incidents are the only record of their existence.

As an outsider looking in and never quite belonging, I shared the trauma, the tears and the laughter of the people who passed through the doors of the Accident and Emergency Department – or the "Cas" as it was known to the residents of the city it served.

The hospital has more than doubled in size since I first started to work there; new buildings and new innovations have made it difficult to keep up with the constant changes in progress. A school of medicine linked to the local university and new medical science blocks have changed the skyline of the city, with further plans in hand to take the hospital into the twenty-first century.

Having no medical qualifications, my duties were of a mundane nature; but being available when I was needed by the staff and knowing the geographical layout of the hospital, I was accepted and indeed welcomed as an extra pair of hands to do the lifting, and an extra pair of legs to run all the errands. Over the years my duties varied. I acted as a receptionist, clerk and porter. I also assisted the nursing staff in the Casualty Department and the fracture clinic, working in the late evening and sometimes throughout the night.

In those early days, it was possible for me to be engaged in those tasks through staff shortage and emergency situations. Now through the changes of administration over the years, and the demarcation lines laid down by the trade unions, it would be very unlikely for any voluntary worker to be allowed to cover such a wide range of duties as I was privileged enough to do. I can say with all honesty that the only time the patients suffered through my services was when they drank my hospital tea!

From the over-crowded area where I first started to work, pushing patients on iron bedsteads, to the various wards and clinics, the Accident and Emergency Department has now blossomed into a modern custom-built area, with the latest equipment and computerised technology. It has an air of clinical efficiency which is most impressive to the observer, but somehow, I still remember with great affection my early days in the department, when the whole of the staff were forced to share the same small building, and were welded into one unit. The lines of communication were short, and a more human approach seemed to be possible when dealing with a wide range of patients.

The ghost still lingers. Perhaps that's why I wrote this book.

Walter Cockshaw

Prologue

The telephone gave one long ring and stopped abruptly. My right hand, holding the cheese sandwich that I had purchased earlier from the dining room, remained poised in the air for a few seconds and proceeded once again in the general direction of my mouth. Why was it, I wondered, that hospital cheese always tasted like soap? Perhaps all large institutions were supplied with a universal compound for multi-purpose use to save money; who knows, the domestic staff could be using it at that moment to scrub the floors. My thoughts strayed into realms of fantasy.

The telephone gave another ring. This time it was longer, and seemed to have a more urgent note. Telephones are not neutral instruments; as soon as you pick up the receiver you are involved with the person at the other end of the wire, or as my friend Sydney says, ensnared by science, so I continued to ignore it.

Whoever was ringing didn't give up easily, it started to ring again and kept on ringing. The sound echoed along the corridor and Claudia, the radiographer on duty, poked her head out of the X-Ray room and saw me sitting in the easy chair that the porters had purloined from the office of one of the consultants. She waved her hand and retired inside again. The wave must have been an indication for me to answer the phone, and I gave a final glance round the area in the hope that one of the porters might have returned, but I could see no one so I picked up the receiver.

'Extension 234.'

'Is that you Danny?' a man's voice enquired.

'No, it's Walter. Danny's on the reception desk relieving the night clerk.'

Danny was the porter in charge of the night shift, and I was at that particular moment sitting in his usual chair and about to drink his tea. There was a pause from the other end, so I sipped my tea and waited.

'This is Ken.' He was one of the missing porters. 'Can you bring the glory wagon to Priest Ward? I've got a client for the Winter Gardens.'

'I'm not sure ...' I began.

'Don't be long. We're on take tonight and Sister may need the bed.'

There was a click as Ken replaced the receiver, leaving me in a fog of indecision and doubt. I had never paid a visit to the Winter Gardens before, and although death was no stranger to me through my war experiences, I had given no thought to the reality of dealing with people who had died in hospital, and I wondered if I had the courage to do it. This was one of the periods when the portering staff were busy dealing with the Saturday night drunks, two overdoses, and helping on the wards, while I was snatching a quick break in between my duties. But there was no point in pondering over the request, as I was not going to pass on this job to anyone. Knowing the procedures from watching the porters, I reached up and took the key for the Winter Gardens from the hook above my chair.

The glory wagon stood in the corner of the basement, half hidden by an office wall, its metal sides reflecting the light from the overhead fluorescent bulb. I steered it into the ever open lift nearby and pressed the button for the first floor. I glanced at the clock on the opposite wall before the gates closed – and it was ten minutes after midnight.

Priest Ward was reserved for the male surgical patients, and it was located halfway along the main hospital corridor. The whole building seemed deserted as I pushed the trolley along, the silence broken only by the purr of rubber wheels and the occasional clatter of the vehicle's lid as it passed over the ridges in the uneven floor.

I stopped outside the ward, parked the conveyance alongside the wall and pushed my way through the swing doors. The ward was lit by a single lamp near the nurses' station, and my appearance caused a flurry of activity as two white-clad figures started pulling the curtains round the beds, and then a folding screen was opened and placed across the ward. This must have been to mask my presence in case some of the patients were still awake. Then a white arm beckoned me onwards. As I turned towards the door again, Ken the porter came through pushing the glory wagon and stopped near the first bed inside the ward. 'Over here,' he whispered quietly, and moving forward he pulled back the curtains and pushed the trolley alongside the bed and opened the top. A white shrouded figure lay on the bed with a label attached, and I approached it with some apprehension. It looked so small in the dim light of the ward and the pathos of the situation struck deep inside of me. 'I'll take the top, you take his feet,' Ken went on. 'And don't for God's sake drop him.'

Together we lifted the silent figure and very gently lowered it on to the tray inside the glory wagon and closed the lid. Trying hard to avoid making any noise, we pushed the vehicle through the doors and back along the corridor, my legs feeling rather weak as I walked. The deaths that I had encountered during the war were, by degree, accepted; war was an unfortunate but sometimes necessary game, the losers paying with their lives. But for me this was a new experience, as dying was channelled into the hospital's system, and dealt with efficiently and according to procedure.

Ken must have noticed my silence.

'Is it the first time you've been to the winter gardens?'

I nodded.

'You'll soon get used to it.'

Get used to what? I thought. I had come to help the living not deal with the dead. We made our way along the corridor to the lift and I pressed the button to take us back down to the basement. As the gates opened at the bottom we eased the wagon out as if to prevent any discomfort to our passenger. The ramp in the basement led to an outside courtyard. The cool night air was like a tonic after the stifling heat of the hospital, and I sucked it in greedily.

The winter gardens were located on the opposite side of the yard, and were fronted by a concrete apron to allow motor vehicles easy access to the building. The darkness outside was only relieved by the glow from the surrounding windows which helped to create strange images from our passing shadows as we crossed the courtyard, but even the gloom could not obscure the large sign on the wall which read "Ring and wait". Ken did neither, but unlocked the door, stepped inside and switched on the lights.

We passed into the inner hall, and there were other doors. One was marked "Private", and another bore the words "Strictly No Admission – Pathology Section". I had no desire to open that one at this hour, so I followed Ken and guided the vehicle through an opening at the end of the hall and into the far room.

On the right-hand side, running along the whole length of the wall, were a series of metal doors that reached from the floor to the ceiling. Each door had four panels and these were numbered consecutively from one to thirty-six. Underneath some of the numbers, names had been chalked, obviously to identify the occupants of the inner chamber, and as Ken opened one I could see the faces inside, pallid and grey-looking, locked in sleep forever.

'This will do,' he said, indicating the empty chamber at the top.

The room had a sweet and sickly smell that I was always to associate with death from that moment on. I gave a shiver, either through the cold air of the surroundings or perhaps my own apprehension, and I felt a sense of shame. As I had volunteered for this work I had better get on with the job, I thought, hoping that Ken had not noticed any reluctance on my part. However, he appeared to be too busy to bother about me. He wheeled the glory wagon over to the lifting device, and between us we placed the shrouded figure on the tray taken from the inner chamber. The device and its passenger were then moved forward, and by a pumping action we brought the tray in line with the top compartment, pushed it inside on to the interior rollers and closed the door.

The recording angel may stand outside the gates of Heaven with a golden book, but all Ken had was a piece of chalk and a ballpoint pen. The chalk to write the name of the man, on the outside panel of the door, and the ballpoint pen to record his details in a book that lay open on a desk in the far corner of the room. From a living, breathing member of the human race a short time ago, our passenger had now become another thread in a web of hospital statistics.

I felt a deep sense of sorrow as Ken locked the door behind us, and as I trundled the trolley across the empty courtyard I felt a lump rising in my throat.

Chapter 1

I Join the W.V.S.

Sydney was already leaning against the bar as I entered the Grand Hotel. He always stood at the end of the counter, and never sat on the stools. When I asked why, he said it was always reassuring to discover that the barmaid had legs that matched the rest of her anatomy.

A glass of bitter stood waiting for me, and I mumbled my thanks before taking the first sip. Sydney and I met regularly every Wednesday lunchtime in the Grand Hotel for about half an hour and had a chat about old times, old friends and the state of the nation in general. We would then say cheerio and depart to our respective jobs.

As I put down my glass, I could sense that Sydney was not his usual self. He seemed quite, and when he fixed me with that baleful stare of his it made me ask:

'Is there something wrong?'

'I didn't know you was a transvestite.'

'I beg your pardon.'

'Transvestite.'

I was not quite sure if it was a question or an accusation; it was always best to play a wait-and-see game with Sydney. He had this characteristic of expressing himself in words that had a wealth of meaning, but only to him, and which had to be interpreted by the person they were directed at. In some cases it was like a secret code, especially when he was chatting to Mary the barmaid. I ordered my round and waited.

'Transvestite,' he repeated, and this time it sounded like an accusation.

'What are you on about?'

‘Fancy you wanting to join the Women’s Voluntary Services!’ he said.

So that was it. I should have guessed the meaning behind his words, and wondered why I had been so stupid as to give his name as a character reference. It was going to be very difficult to explain to a person like Sydney, then again I had never expected my background to be checked by any organisation. Not that I had anything to hide, but I judged myself to be a paragon of all the virtues in my social life, and I was surprised that other people had not reached the same conclusions.

I think I had better explain. It all started in the Autumn of 1974, when my car had to go in to the garage for a service, and for the first time in many years I had to travel by bus. I joined the queue at the local bus stop, and greeted them all with a cheery ‘good morning’, and I was greeted with a grunt from the man in front of me, and curious stares from the rest of the group. I felt like a gatecrasher at a party as they chatted amongst themselves and completely ignored me. The conversation that ensued between some of the women was not very inspiring for a Monday morning; topics like the weather, the previous night’s T.V. programmes, the sorry state of Betty in the wages office, and was George in the accounts department going to do the right thing by her?

When the bus finally arrived it was a double-decker and I was taken by surprise. Although I was halfway down the queue I was new at the game, and I was the last to get on. It was one of those older type vehicles with a rear entrance, and just inside there were two long seats facing each other. It was the period when all buses actually had conductors, and this one barred my way to prevent me going upstairs, and with a sweep of his arm directed me inside. The only seat available was between two stout ladies, and the very thought of sitting and facing the four passengers opposite did not appeal to me at all. I always get embarrassed in situations like that, so I stood up and clutched the overhead rail to steady me.

The conductor had other ideas, however, when he came round to collect his fares. He wasn't in a very good mood, I think his wife must have had a headache the night before, and there was a nasty growl in his voice.

'There's a seat behind you. Sit down!'

I obeyed weakly; I could sense the iron in the soul of the man. I sat down, I wasn't going to argue. Four pairs of eyes now directed their gaze in my direction from the opposite seat and I felt most uncomfortable. I wondered if I had used too much of my new Masterman aftershave, or if I had left my zip unfastened. I had an urge to find out, but thought better of it. Moving my hand in that direction on a public transport vehicle could be dangerous. Men have gone to prison for less.

Avoiding looking directly opposite at my fellow passengers was difficult because seated in line with me was a young lady wearing what can only be described as a micro skirt, it was too short to be a mini. She was a very pretty girl, and I tried in vain to avoid looking at her over-exposed legs. I kept turning my head right and left, and up and down, to avert my eyes, and the other passengers must have thought I was suffering from St. Vitus Dance, or some strange nervous disease. The girl must have senses my embarrassment because she moved her handbag from her side and used it as a kind of chastity belt, and I was somewhat relieved by her action.

Turning my eyes upward over her head to avoid eye-to-eye confrontation, I noticed the poster stuck in the window of the bus. Printed on a white background was a blue hand with its fingers outstretched, but whoever designed it had got the format all wrong. It looked as if some monster from outer space was giving a "V" sign to us poor earthlings. Then I noticed the text underneath it which read “Lend a Helping Hand. Ring or Call at the Voluntary Workers Bureau”. This was followed by a telephone number and an address. It was to be several weeks before I took the advice printed on the poster, but it was from such a chance beginning that I got involved in voluntary work that in some ways changed my life.

Christmas was rapidly approaching, and I contemplated with dismay the tinsel and plastic facade that shrouds the festive season. Perhaps I was a pessimist but I always felt sad and depressed on this occasion. It wasn’t that I lacked invitations from my family and friends, but the whole event seemed false and remote from the real meaning of the word Christmas. It was when I was deliberating one day on this subject that I thought of the poster. Couldn’t I do something different this year, I mused, like working in a hospital? Surely I could fit in somewhere as a volunteer worker. And I was caught in a wave of enthusiasm. The telephone directory provided me with the address and phone number of the Voluntary Workers Bureau, so I rang for an appointment.

The lady who answered the phone sounded quite young and had a pleasant manner. I told her who I was and what I wanted to do, and she listened patiently.

‘Why not come and see us one night?’ she went on, ‘I’m sure we can help you.’

‘Thank you, I will do,’ I replied. At last I was on my way.

* * *

I found the entrance to the Voluntary Workers Bureau in a building along a small alley opposite the railway station. They shared the premises, according to the nameplates outside, with offices for the family planning clinic, the single parent families, and some charity called Save the Children. I did a quick mental permutation with the names and wondered why they didn't amalgamate and save money. Making my way to the second floor I found the door marked Voluntary Services and, obeying the instructions, I knocked and walked in. Seated at a desk with her back to the window was a slim blonde lady, very pretty, and young in appearance. She raised her head from what seemed to be a pile of paperwork and gave me a warm smile.

'Hello, can I help you?' she asked.

She certainly could, but I thought I had better confine myself to the purpose of my visit, so I explained who I was and why I was there.

'Of course, Mr Cockshaw, I have your enquiry here. You want to do some voluntary work at Christmas. Could you give me some personal details?'

It took quite a time and a cup of coffee to pour out part of my life history. She seemed quite interested in the details of my army career, how I nearly captured Field Marshal Rommel in the Western Desert during the war, and even the fact that I had done some amateur acting, even though the characters were mostly butlers and undertakers. She may have thought those could be useful if I was to be let loose on the hospital wards. She wrote all my details down on the writing pad that she had on her desk and then she looked up.

'I see that you live in the south of the city. The Royal is the nearest hospital to you, but they are very particular about voluntary workers. We do, however, meet with the chief nursing officer from time to time, so we'll mention your offer to her.'

The young blonde and I parted good friends, and she promised that I would be hearing from her or the hospital in the near future.

After my interview the days slipped by and the anticipated letter did not arrive. To some degree this was a blow to my ego; here was I offering my services free to the medical profession, and there was no one wanting to take advantage of my gesture. Obviously the news had not yet permeated through to the Regional Health Board, or to the higher echelons of the B.M.A. However, I must be patient, the mad scramble for my services would no doubt come later.

It did.

Well it was not exactly a mad scramble, but a letter that came by second-class post from the assistant chief nursing officer (I suppose the chief nursing officer must have been on holiday at that time). It requested me to phone and make an appointment to come and see her regarding my application. Why anyone should want to interview me for wanting to work without pay puzzled me; wasn't I eminently acceptable? Surely with my background I should be taken at face value alone, and she must have my details from the Voluntary Workers Bureau. But as Sydney said later, the hospital board had to be careful, they probably had too many bloody idiots working for them already without adding to their number.

Why is it that I get my ideas all twisted? Perhaps being brought up on a diet of Charles Dickens and other Victorian novelists that had helped to colour my imagination. The assistant chief nursing officer who now sat opposite me bore no resemblance to Sarah Gamp, she did not wear a blood-stained apron or have a gin bottle within reach, and I very much doubt if she imbibed any liquid stronger than tea. She was dressed in a smart blue uniform with white facings, and the warmth of her greeting immediately put me at ease; it was only afterwards that I realised how naive I had been to think that I – a complete outsider with no medical experience – might be allowed to work in a large general hospital without being assessed.

It was when the smile on her face slowly faded that the questions started.

'Why do you want to do voluntary work in a hospital, Mr Cockshaw? I gather from your background that you could direct your efforts into other channels where they would be more appreciated?'

It was not a good start. I tried to think of an answer that would perhaps relay my feelings, but it was hard to express how I felt.

'Well ... er ... I just thought I could help.'

'But you have no medical qualifications.'

I admitted the fact.

'We have a responsibility to all our patients.'

'I realise that.'

'Under no circumstances do we allow any voluntary workers to become involved in the treatment of any of our patients.'

'Yes, of course.'

'That leaves only the menial duties ...'

'Well ... Yes.'

'... and we *have* a good ancillary staff.'

'Well there must be some work I can do?'

'What, for instance?'

'Well,' I burst out. 'Empty the bed pans, help wash the patients, serve the meals, run the errands ...'

'You'll get no thanks.'

'I don't want any thanks. I had a strange idea that I might be useful to someone, somewhere in this hospital, if not the staff, perhaps the patients; but I'm evidently wrong.'

I was now prepared to accept defeat. I thought it was time for me to go. My hospital career seemed to have ended before it had even started. I could have crawled under the door, I felt so small.

It was then that the assistant chief nursing officer smiled, that warm engaging smile she had greeted me with when I first arrived. She stood up and walked from behind her desk.

'I think that we both understand each other now, Mr Cockshaw.' she said. 'Welcome to the Royal Hospital, we would be very pleased if you could spare some time to help us over the Christmas holidays. If you will follow me I will show you the areas where you may be needed.'

As I trailed meekly behind her she led me through various wards and finally we crossed a bridge over a busy main road that linked the main hospital to a smaller building. A large sign on the wall with an arrow above it read "Accident and Emergency Department". Along a corridor we turned a corner, and soon we were facing a lapping tide of humanity. People were sitting on chairs, lying on trolleys, or dashing about trying to get the attention of the nursing staff. We stood there for some time before the assistant chief nursing officer managed to attract the attention of the male charge nurse and told him who I was, and my desire to help over the Christmas period. 'Why wait for Christmas?' he said as he stopped to grab an X-ray plate from a passing porter. 'It's Christmas every day of the year in this place, we could do with your help now.'

I found it difficult to understand my own motives for this urge to work as a volunteer. Was it to help people in need, or to help rescue my own soul from boredom and loneliness? The truth lies probably between the two, but before the scheduled three week starting date, I found myself actively employed both on the wards and in the Accident and Emergency department, or the "Cas" to use its popular name.

Life would never be quite the same again.

* * *

It was several weeks after I had started my voluntary work that the letter arrived. It was in a buff coloured envelope and stamped on the outside in large letters were the words

"Women's Voluntary Services". I checked the address to make sure it had been delivered to the right house, but yes it had, and my name was on the front. Overcome by curiosity, I opened it and extracted the letter which was headed "Dear Sir" and seemed quite genuine. It could hardly be one of Sydney's little jokes, so I read on.

"Dear Sir,

We note that you are in regular attendance at the Accident and Emergency Department of the Royal Hospital as a voluntary worker and that you do not belong to any organised body recognised by the hospital authorities. It would be desirable both from the hospital's point of view and your own that you should be working under the cloak of some recognised organisation so that you may be covered by some form of insurance, and be noted as an official worker. You would then be conforming to a code of ethics relating to conduct and confidentiality, which I am sure you agree is most desirable in this kind of work.

The Women's Voluntary Services can provide you with this cover, and if you would call at the above address, at your liberty, we would gladly welcome you in our ranks.

Sincerely Yours,

Cynthia Pushbutton (Mrs)
City Organiser."

My first reaction on reading the letter was one of amusement. It must be a joke, I thought, I'll ignore it. But then again the envelope and the letter heading looked genuine enough, and it was hardly likely that anyone would go to such devious lengths to play such a joke on me. There was only one thing to do in a situation like this, so I did it. I reached for the phone, dialled the number that was on the letter and waited. After a few seconds a woman's voice answered.

'Women's Voluntary Services.'

'May I speak with Mrs Pushbutton please.'

'Hold on please, I'll fetch her.'

Well, she did exist then. I waited for some time before a breathless voice answered me.

'Cynthia Pushbutton, sorry to keep you waiting, I was down in the basement sorting out blankets for the air disaster.'

'Air disaster!'

'It should be a good show. It's only an exercise, of course, but one never knows, does one? What can I do for you?'

'My name's Walter Cockshaw. You wrote to me about joining the W.V.S.'

'Oh yes, I remember.'

'Forgive me, I'm a little confused.'

'Confused?'

'I never knew that you had male members in your organisation.'

'Oh yes, we have a few.'

I was even more perplexed. Male members in the W.V.S? I would be a man in a woman's world! I sat clutching the receiver.

'Are you still there?'

'Er ... yes.'

'Well, do come along and see us, we would like to get you signed up and make it official, there's no need to make an appointment. Pop in any time. Thank you for phoning. Goodbye.'

'Goodbye.' But the line was dead.

It must be easier for a camel to pass through the eye of a needle than to become a member of the Women's Voluntary

Services. A converted house in the city centre acted as the headquarters for the organisation, and I duly entered through the door marked "Enquiries" and passed into the ground floor office. Sitting on a chair squeezed in between two desks was a middle-aged lady busily knitting a shapeless garment that spilled over onto the floor alongside the various balls of wool she was using. To my inexperienced eye it looked a tangled mess, but to her it must have been a labour of love, as this masterpiece commanded the whole of her attention.

In spite of my discreet cough she continued to ignore me and went on knitting to a rhythm of words that sounded like 'Quick ... slow ... Quick ... quick ... slow ...' Her fingers kept in time with her mouth. Here was a veritable Victor Silvester of the knitting world, and as I watched her I half expected her to get up and do a fox-trot round the office floor, until I noticed what must have been a pair of size nine bootees on her feet. After another arm swinging movement, and a further six bars of 'Quick ... quick ... slow ...', she looked up from her knitting.

'Sorry to keep you waiting,' she said. 'I had to get that row finished. Can I help you?'

'Mrs Pushbutton?' I asked.

Her face froze a little.

'Oh, you want the city crowd, we are the county group.'

She stressed the last five words as if to leave me in no doubt as to the superior status of the county branch. She picked up her knitting again, leaving me standing there and no wiser as to the location of the lady I had come to see. I stood for a moment wondering what to do, then a voice which obviously meant that I was dismissed snapped out: 'Upstairs and on the left!' The 'Quick ... quick ... slow...' faded away as I climbed upwards and, discovering the only door on the left-hand side of the corridor, I knocked loudly on the panel. A sharp 'Come in' came from the other side. I pushed my way in and was met by a cloud of white vapour that filled the room, limiting my vision to the shadowy images of a desk, a chair and several more obscure shapes, but nothing that resembled a human form.

'Mrs Pushbutton?' I shouted in an alarmed voice.

A large figure loomed up from below the desk. It was holding a teapot.

'I was trying to make myself a lunchtime cup of tea,' a female voice said. 'But I can't switch the kettle off.'

I moved over to her through the steam that was now condensing on the windows and located the cause of the panic. Bending down, I managed to switch off the kettle and the room slowly cleared to reveal the figure of a large lady who started pouring water into the teapot she was still carrying.

'I do like a good cup of tea,' she went on. 'I don't like these tea-bags really, but we have to use them, as I never know where to put the tea leaves.' I was glad Sydney wasn't there to tell her.

A cup of tea and ten minutes later, I established that I was talking to *THE* Mrs Pushbutton and managed to tell her the reason for my visit.

'Oh yes, I remember, you wanted to join the W.V.S.'

'No, *you* asked me to join. You sent me a letter.'

'That's right, I'll look you up in the files.'

She moved over to a cabinet and started looking through a group of folders.

'What did you say your name was?'

'Cockshaw. Walter Cockshaw.'

'Oh yes, you will be under P.'

'No, C for Cockshaw.'

'No, P for Pending.'

She returned to the desk with a folder in her hand, and I gave a sigh as once again she requested details of my background. I must admit she didn't look at my teeth or demand my parents' marriage certificate, but the questions were somewhat searching, and I had to stop and think before answering. But on the whole all went well until she asked for the names of two people who would give me a reference. This stopped me in my tracks. First of all, I was surprised to think that anyone would doubt my integrity by making such a request, and secondly I could never think of the addresses of people I knew who would vouch for me to prove that I was an honest and upright member of society. I wracked my brains for a time.

'Would my employers do for one?'

'They would indeed.'

After delving again into my memory I realised that I knew Sydney's address. I couldn't very well forget it. He called his cottage The Old Ruin and claimed he'd named it after his wife. Perhaps he would give me a reference. So I took a chance and gave his name to Mrs Pushbutton. That completed the session. The ordeal was over and Mrs Pushbutton seemed satisfied. All being well, I was now enlisted in the ranks of the opposite sex. I had struck a blow for male emancipation; I had no bra to burn, but I could set fire to my braces. I thought better of it as I only had one pair.

The news of my final acceptance as a member of the W.V.S. must have echoed along the corridors of power and reached the highest personage in the land, and though I can't possibly take all the credit, that Great Lady (who shall be nameless) in her wisdom granted a Royal Charger sometime afterwards, turning the Women's Voluntary Services into The Women's Royal Voluntary Services. A splendid tribute to the members past and present. I really did try and explain to Sydney why I'd joined the W.R.V.S. but I didn't have much success.

'I thought they did meals on wheels,' he said.

'They do.'

'If you get near them it will be squeals on wheels.'

You can't reason with people like Sydney.

Chapter 2

The Hospital

The hospital stood near the centre of the city, but when it first opened its doors in 1771 it was surrounded by green fields, and described as "standing on a salubrious eminence, and occupying [together with close and gardens] about eight acres of land". The initial project was funded by private subscriptions, but from the very beginning it was advertised as being "open for the sick, lame, and poor of any county or nation". But in practice, apart from accident cases, patients had to have a letter of recommendation from a subscriber.

During those early years the hospital gardens yielded fruit and vegetables, and a herd of cows produced milk for the patients and staff. Being employed as a porter depended on one's ability to brew beer, look after the cattle, and having a knowledge of gardening, all for the princely wage of twenty-five pounds a year!

Now, when viewed from the outside, the old part of the hospital looked like a motley collection of buildings that were thrown together without thought or reason. In spite of the constant changes that were always taking place, the hospital never seemed quite adequate for the growing city it served. The original buildings had over the years been extended in all directions, swallowing up streets of Victorian houses, bestriding the main roads with overhead bridges and underground corridors to join the scattered wards and departments. The old part of the exterior had a grey look, caused by the accumulated dirt and the passing traffic, and this facade contrasted strangely with the concrete and glass of the newly built tower blocks that had been added.

To walk through the corridors in the original part of the hospital was like stepping back in time. Portraits of long-departed doctors and surgeons and stern-faced matrons frowned down from the walls at the groups of laughing nurses as they passed, oblivious of the disapproval of these ghosts from the past. Two large grandfather clocks stood on guard at opposite ends of the corridor, their wooden cases carved with the names of the surgeons who had dedicated their lives to the service of the people of the city. Their mellow tones as they chimed the hours away had a reverent sound, as if to mark the passing of the benefactors who had donated them.

Time had had little effect on the spirit of the hospital. It had helped withstand the onslaught of plagues and pestilence for nearly two and a half centuries. It had opened its doors to the victims of many wars, and stood as a symbol of help to the sick. Old prints and photographs reflected scenes from the past, surgeons dressed in frock coats, nurses in ankle-length uniforms, and wards heated by a single coal stove. Engraved tablets on the wall over some of the beds recorded the names of the people and the various societies that had endowed them; even some of the older wards bore the names of the more important benefactors. In the past the people of the city maintained the hospital by public subscription, and even the workers contributed pennies from their meagre pay packets. It was a place that everyone could turn to in their hour of need irrespective of position and class.

The hospital had a soul of its own. Passing through the doors of the main entrance the visitors were enveloped by the prevailing atmosphere. For all its faults, this place was dear to the hearts of the people, it had served their families over the years, tried to cure their ills, or let its patients die in dignity.

In spite of having roots in the past, the hospital also had a stake in the future. A medical school was now a part of the local university, and the students trailed after the consultants as they did their rounds of the hospital wards. New departments sprang up that had strange sounding names, and the terms of reference for the staff also altered, making it difficult at times to assess their true position in the scheme of things, and even more difficult to know how to address them by using their correct titles. One knew the pecking order of pupil nurses, student nurses, state enrolled nurses, state registered nurses, sisters and charge nurses, but beyond that, alas the matrons had now vanished and senior nursing officers of all degrees were now in charge. The old order had changed, and even the patients who were always eager to acknowledge the status of the person that was attending them were often at a loss.

But the hospital was always there for the people of the city to use and sometimes abuse. A haven in times of illness, and always open for the sick, lame and poor just as it had been 250 years ago.

Chapter 3

The Volunteer's Bible

There must be many reasons why some people want to work as unpaid helpers in a hospital. It must fulfil some need in their lives, perhaps helping to combat boredom or loneliness, or it may be a desire for some form of social contact, or joy through work. Others may regard their efforts as a community duty, a form of self flagellation that is good for the soul. It could be likened to the man who was asked why he was banging his head against the wall. He replied that it was a lovely feeling when he stopped. Some may even think it may enhance their reputation, and use it as a status symbol, to give an impression of social usefulness to their friends.

Some volunteers are motivated from purely Christian principles, and give their time and energy to help people. It is unfortunate that even in this group, as in others, a lot of good work can be undermined by some over-zealous individuals who insist in offering prayers instead of bedpans. One such person, known as Holy Joe, would start to pray for the patients at the slightest excuse. He was also a faith healer, and he offered to help the patients on the ward where he worked by the laying on of hands. Most of them were short-stay cases who had been admitted for routine operations, and Joe's promise of Heaven must have been sheer Hell for them. When he put in an appearance they either pretended to be asleep or, if they could get out of bed, made a dash for the toilet. He prayed with so much fervour that most of them thought they were ready to shuffle off this mortal coil. He offered religious comfort like a priest administering the last rites, and strangely enough his activities escaped the notice of the busy staff for quite a time.

His departure was hastened by a visiting doctor whom he assumed to be a new patient, and when he offered his services as a faith healer, the doctor had to be restrained from laying his hands on Joe.

Other organisations such as the Red Cross and the St. John's Ambulance Brigade also supplied volunteers who did work which complemented the efforts of the permanent staff, but as most of their training did not relate to hospital procedures, it was only the nursing staff who treated the patients, and first-aid stopped at the front door. It is hard for some voluntary workers to realise that they have no status within the hospital where they work, and their services may be resented, or just tolerated, unless a bridge of understanding is built up between the volunteer and the staff they work with. Voluntary workers should never exceed their duties. It is a known fact that in every casualty department throughout the land, the nursing staff, and the porters, think that they can diagnose every kind of illness and injury before the doctors ever see their patients. And strangely enough they are often right. Over a period of time these same attitudes could be adopted by some of the voluntary workers, and this could lead to potentially dangerous situations. It was only the doctors and the trained staff that dealt with the medical problems of the patients, and it was only under their direction that the volunteers worked. Mistakes by the permanent staff may be excusable, but a mistake by a voluntary worker is unforgivable, as it may destroy the good will that has been built up over a number of years. But in spite of erring on the side of caution, it was still very easy for the unwary to get involved in medical procedures.

One busy Saturday night I relieved the nurse acting as the doctor's receptionist for the minor cases, or the walking wounded, as they were known to the staff. The duties were relatively simple, and consisted of calling the patients from the waiting room to see the doctor and afterwards directing them for their specific treatment, X-rays, etc. according to the instructions written on their casualty cards.

After the casualty officer had seen about a dozen patients, he came out of his consulting room followed by a woman clutching her treatment card.

'I'm going for supper now,' he said. 'I'll see the other patients when I get back. I've been on duty now for eight hours without a break, I must go for a meal ... Oh by the way, look after this lady.' He indicated the woman behind him, and strode off along the corridor before I could reply.

I took the treatment card from the patient's hand to enter the details in the record book, but the doctor's writing was so atrocious in parts that it was impossible to read it all. It has always been a contention of mine that certain groups who deal with the public should have lessons in the art of handwriting, and top of the list would be members of the medical profession. Why they can't write plainly is beyond me; a wrong interpretation of what they have written could have dire consequences for some of their unfortunate patients.

My particular doctor must have been in a hurry to go for his supper, and I thought it best not to bleep him. He would not be pleased. I made my way to the sister in charge and handed her the card.

'Can you tell me what treatment the doctor has ordered for this patient, Sister?'

She studied it for a moment. 'You'd better go and ask him,' she replied.

'I can't he's gone for his supper. I don't want to keep the patient waiting.'

She looked at it again. 'That word looks like X-ray, it can't be anything else.'

'But he's not filled in an X-ray form.'

‘Well, you make one out.’

She turned her attention to the patient she was dealing with; I was obviously dismissed. I stood bewildered for a while, but she was in charge and who was I to question her decision? I had never filled in an X-ray form before, and as the patient had been complaining about her very stiff neck, I just wrote on the card “X-ray neck” and signed it Walter Cockshaw, then I directed her to the X-ray Department and crossed my fingers that the radiographer would not phone the Casualty Department to find out who Doctor Cockshaw was.

However, it evidently did the trick; she returned after about twenty minutes with an envelope containing her X-ray plates, which I put on the doctor’s desk to await his return.

When he did come back he looked grim-faced as though he had been dining off hospital chips, which were not conducive to a man’s well-being after a long spell on duty. He picked up the woman’s casualty card and then her X-ray plates. He turned to me with a puzzled look on his face.

‘I didn’t order this woman to be X-rayed. Who sent her?’

This was a situation in which I was not going to win. I could not tell him that Sister had instructed me to send the patient. Either way I was not going to be very popular.

‘I sent her, Doctor.’

‘Why?’

I pointed to the writing on the card. ‘I thought that word was X-ray so I filled a form in and sent her.’

‘I’m the one who determines if a patient wants an X-ray, not you.’ He pointed to the card. ‘That word is “rest” not X-ray.’

‘I’m sorry, Doctor. I’ll send the lady home, she’s been here a long time.’

Thankful that the ordeal was over and I had got away lightly, I made my escape from the consulting room, and started filling the patient's details in the record book when the doctor came out of his room with the X-ray plates in his hand.

'Has that lady gone home yet?'

'No she's still in the waiting room.'

'Bring her back, I want to see her.'

I duly ushered the woman back into the consulting room, and made for the door.

'Don't go away, I want you to take this lady to the treatment room,' the doctor said.

One hour and about 20 patients later I saw the woman getting into a taxi, her neck encased in a large collar that reached almost to her ears. She would never know that she had me to thank – or curse – for the treatment that she had just received. Which of course brings me back to the moral of this story: never exceed your duties as a voluntary worker, but encourage the nursing staff to exceed theirs for the welfare of the patients.

Any volunteer who works within the framework of a hospital soon recognises the snares and pitfalls when it comes to working in harmony with the staff. There is always to some degree a conflict of temperament between people who work in close proximity, and it is very hard to remain aloof when disagreements occur. The cowardly way out is to agree with everyone all the time, and although this will probably earmark you as a creeper without a mind of your own, it could help you to avoid any repercussions.

The efficiency of any Casualty Department can be assessed by the way the tea is made and distributed, and the voluntary worker should always accept a cup when it is offered. At the Royal, tea-making methods were usually highly organised, and in some cases quite unofficial. Protocol played a large part, and the student and pupil nurses did not have to be told whose duty it was to make a pot of tea, unless of course I was at hand. It was quite noticeable how the staff could go without a meal break when working under pressure, but depended on a quick cup of tea to revitalise them. A complicated inter-change took place during the very busy periods which allowed everyone in turn to partake of a cuppa.

The word tea was never mentioned openly in front of the patients in the Casualty Department in my early days, owing to some of them having to wait for long periods before seeing the doctor. The only source of refreshment was from a machine in the waiting room that dispensed liquids claiming to be tea, coffee or soup, according to which button you pressed, and there was a notice above it warning patients not to use it before they saw a doctor. This was not to avoid any toxic effect from the beverage, but to lessen any waiting time in case a general anaesthetic had to be administered.

To avoid riots from our thirsty patients who might see us drinking, the staff used a code name to mask the word 'tea'. It was not unusual for a nurse to approach a colleague to tell her to fetch the T.C.P. or that the medicine in the dispensary was waiting. One student nurse was told to go and get Rosie Lee, so she went to another department to find a Chinese nurse of the same name and who didn't think it very funny at the time.

To be offered tea by the staff was a gesture of acceptance and it could never be refused. It was a proud moment in my life when the porters offered me a cup, as I knew then that I had penetrated the upper strata of the hospital workers to be accorded such an honour. Soon afterwards successive shifts of the nursing staff and the receptionists also asked me to share their brew, and I always accepted with profound thanks, not wanting to scorn this ancient rite of friendship.

It would be wrong of me to give the impression that life in the Casualty Department was one long orgy of tea drinking. It only seemed like it, as the hours I worked covered the change-over period of the nursing staff, the receptionists and the porters, all with their own means of making a "brew-up" in which I was invited to share.

The infernal machine in the waiting room that also dispensed hot drinks was not very reliable. To make it work one had to kick the left-hand side panel very hard, after putting the required amount of coins in. If the front was kicked it dispensed an empty cup and a gurgle, but the severe blow on the side inspired it to pour forth a hot liquid that was not always a cup of tea; sometimes it was chocolate instead. It was only possible to tell the difference when you drank it – the chocolate looked like muddy water, the tea tasted like it.

The volunteer therefore never refused tea, as apart from causing offence to the person who made it, the gesture might not be repeated in the future. So a general rule was: accept all the tea that is offered, and if none is forthcoming take a hint – change your toilet soap or change your job.

After drinking all the tea that's about, the voluntary worker should know the exact location of the nearest loo.

Chapter 4

The Porters

"... Oh Mr Porter what shall I do? You've taken me to X-ray and I want to use the loo. Take me back to Casualty as quickly as you can. Oh Mr Porter, you are a silly man."

Danny the porter was breathing hard as he slumped down in his chair and reached for his mug of tea. 'It's always the same,' he went on. 'Every time I take a patient to X-ray they decide they want to go for a piss, so I have to push them back to Casualty. There must be something in that X-ray department that affects their kidneys.'

Moving patients from place to place was one of the main duties of the porters. It was very hard on the feet after they had been on duty for a few hours, so the odd grumble was understandable.

The porters came in all sorts of shapes and sizes. Some were quite young, while others had spent a lifetime in the service of the hospital. They came from mixed backgrounds, and unfortunately some of the staff seriously underestimated their abilities – taking the view that the porters' intelligence status was below average, or they would not be doing that type of work, which was far from the truth. Many did the work rather than sign on the dole during periods of depression. One porter, who was a brilliant artist who had exhibited at the Royal Academy, worked at the hospital because the hours suited him, and allowed him time to continue with his art studies. During the summer vacations, many university students, some studying medicine, joined the portering staff as temporary workers, and a student of theology, known as the Bishop, came to widen his knowledge of life by working in the Accident and Emergency Department.

Military historians have written about battles being won through having good lines of communications and supplies, and in some ways the efficiency of a hospital can be judged by the same principles. It was certainly the case with the porters in the Casualty Department that I worked with. This particular group were on rotating eight-hour shifts, and they provided cover for the Department for 24 hours a day. There were four shifts of eight porters, which made it possible for one group to have every fourth week off duty. These shifts, however, rarely had a full complement of porters owing to sickness and holidays, and it was through such situations arising that I was made more than welcome when I appeared on the scene.

Before the appointment of hospital security officers, the porters in the Casualty Department were called upon to deal with all the major and minor incidents that arose in the hospital. They chased unwanted intruders out of the wards and from the nearby nurses' home. They restrained violent patients, pacified the drunks when they got out of hand, and detained would-be thieves until the police took over. They were the hospital's Jack-of-all-Trades. When equipment or machinery broke down during the night they would somehow manage in difficult situations to keep the place ticking over until help arrived. Very often they broke the hospital's regulations in dealing with such incidents, but necessity overruled these laws.

In the hospital's early days the status of the porters was very low. The staff dining room was closed to them, and they were expected to have their meals in any convenient corner so long as they were out of sight. Yet in spite of the strict pecking order for the staff, on the whole the relationship between the porters, the medical and the nursing staff was very good, and this was perhaps due to the fact that they all worked in close proximity to each other. This was to change in later years with a move to a new Casualty Department as the hospital extended.

The mode of communication with the porters was for any member of the nursing staff to yell in a loud voice along the corridor "Porter! Porter!". This method did not always evoke the best response from some of the porters, especially when one particular staff nurse known as 'Big Gob' was on duty. They would give me a nudge and yell back "The Pox Doctor's on his way, he'll look after you." They knew it annoyed her as she was a stickler for protocol, always addressing me as Mr Cockshaw and insisting that everyone should do the same.

The way of transporting patients to the wards in those early days was by iron bedsteads that were lined up in the corridor opposite the cubicles. These monsters rattled along the corridors and in and out of the lifts, jarring the patients, in spite of our efforts to smooth their passage. We did at times have to move at great speeds to get a patient who was critically ill to the operating theatre, or to the intensive care unit, often leaving the nurse or doctor who was with us chasing at our heels. It was a great relief when these flying bedsteads were slowly phased out, and the introduction of more trolleys in the casualty department helped made conditions easier for both the patients and the staff.

The porters had their own names for people and places. In the beginning it was not always easy for the others to accept me in my role as a voluntary worker, and my first appearance on the scene inspired the remark: "Here comes the Pox Doctor's Clerk." But as the weeks passed and I was assessed by each successive shift, I was soon accepted. I discovered that the mortuary was known as the winter gardens, and the metal coffin on wheels which was used to collect the dead from the wards was called the glory wagon.

I soon found my way around the hospital without getting lost. I learnt how to undress injured patients without causing them further distress, and gave a hand in removing the dead from the wards. It was hard going at times, especially dealing with some of the patients known as 'N.F.As' – people with no fixed abode. This was always a testing time, removing clothes that had been worn for weeks (perhaps months) and finding underwear and socks that had rotted on their bodies, and which disintegrated at the touch. This proved to be so nauseating that it made me wonder why I'd ever started doing this work. Then of course there were the fleas and lice to deal with.

Unfortunately fleas are no respecters of persons, and in spite of the barrier clothing these tiny immigrants crossed the demarcation lines and travelled home with members of the staff. The porters were often called to help bathe some of these homeless patients if they were being sent to a ward, a task not willingly accepted but always carried out, to prevent the nurse who was looking after the patient being left alone with some undesirable character. The bath water would at times turn from a black colour to a light grey as it was constantly changed. I often wondered if their last bath had been administered by the midwife at their birth. Although water helped remove some of the dirt, the odour still remained; the cloying stink from torso and feet permeated the masks we sometimes wore, and seemed to be absorbed by our own clothing for hours afterwards.

Perhaps it was because I did not try to escape the distasteful duties that I was accepted by the porters. They shared their tea with me, and told me their latest batch of lewd jokes, while the Bishop, who would sometimes be present, would give a wry smile and bury his head in the book he was reading.

George, who was the oldest member of the Porters' Lodge and who had spent most of his life in the service of the hospital, would regale all the newcomers with horror stories from the past.

'You don't know how well off you are these days,' he would say. 'I remember before the war we had a flu epidemic one year, and people were dying like flies. We only had a small mortuary in those days, and it was so full that we used to stack the bodies criss-crossed on top of each other in the only space available behind the door. We also had to make sure that we left a window open when we locked up at night.'

'Was that to let the smell out?' someone would ask.

'No. When the bodies at the bottom of the pile softened up the bloody lot would fall over and block the doorway, so we had to climb in through the window to move them.'

As the years passed there were romances between the porters and the nursing staff that led to marriages. There were heartaches too, through illness and death, that affected the lives of the people I was involved with, and made me realise that even hospital staff are mortal. We had our black sheep too. One porter was caught, while working on the night-shift, loading some hospital linen into his car, and a later search of his house by the police revealed a veritable mountain of stolen blankets, sheets and pillows.

* * *

Hospital life also had its moments of humour. We visited the wards to help lift overweight patients back into their beds, an operation that sometimes needed four porters, as some of the people who needed lifting weighed over twenty-stone. One such patient was so huge he was known as Mount Everest to the staff. He had a heart condition, and when he was rushed in for treatment, his body oozed over both sides of the trolley, making it impossible for us to raise the sides. He was obviously very ill, and as we struggled to get him in the lift, Ken the porter, who was a small dapper man, turned and whispered in my ear.

'Bloody hell, Walter, let's get him to the ward quick. I'm off duty soon, and if he snuffs it I don't want the job of squeezing him in the fridge in the winter gardens!'

Ken had scant respect for authority, but the patients who got to know him all loved him, as he added some colour to their lives. If Sister was missing he would often lead a crocodile of porters and nurses around a ward banging a metal bedpan and singing "Come and join us". One of his specialities was a song and dance act, and when he had finished performing it one day the nursing officer, alerted by the noise, appeared on the scene.

'Was that you singing?' she asked.

'Who did you think it was?' Ken replied. 'You can't get Frank Sinatra on the National Health.'

Before the computer era at the hospital, all the Casualty patients were booked in on a hand-written casualty card which was handed to the staff. The patient's surname was always written first, followed by their other names. Thus when they were called from the waiting room, the name Smith John was reversed to become John Smith. The porters, always game for a laugh, would often make up cards for mythical patients and add them to the pile. The nurse on duty, usually one of the students, would find herself in a crowded waiting room shouting for non-existent patients with names like Ivor Biggun, Mustapha Shite, Willie Havit and Ivor Payne, just to name a few. The poor nurse could not understand the ensuing laughter that greeted her call, and wondered where her patient had disappeared to, while the porters in the background enjoyed her embarrassment. The sisters on duty, however, did not find these episodes amusing, and directed some strong, unlady-like language at the porters responsible.

One of the members of the portering staff was Jock, an exile from his native city of Glasgow, and known to his colleagues as the Porridge Gobbler. He was a big burly man, and he told many tales of the past fights that he had been involved in. By his manner it was easy to visualise him brawling outside some bar on a Saturday night, as he was quick-tempered and easy to offend. But despite these shortcomings he had a natural sense of humour.

Jock, in common with some of the other porters, had a great dislike for certain members of the staff. Amongst them was a Nigerian who worked in the hospital kitchens whom he always addressed as Sambo, and whenever they met they exchanged insults. One Saturday evening, between the patients' supper time and visiting time, Jock and I were pushing the glory wagon along the hospital corridor after collecting a body from a male surgical ward to take to the winter gardens, when Sambo loomed into sight pushing a food trolley. Seeing Jock, he stopped, leaned on his vehicle and said after a pause:

'Who you got 'dere Jock? One of your victims?'

'No, Sambo, one of yours. You've poisoned him with that bloody food you serve up.'

'Ah, the poor man was unlucky to have died in this place.'

'Unlucky,' said Jock. 'It was his good fortune. If he had died in Nigeria you would be having him for breakfast.'

We walked on out of earshot before Sambo could think of an answer.

New members of the portering staff were also victims of their colleagues' sense of humour. Some were sent to the theatres for bone nails, to the pharmacy for flasks of super wet water and to pick up some blue blood for a member of the aristocracy from the haematology department.

One Saturday night I was donning a white coat when I was approached by a tall, good-looking porter I had never seen before. He came forward, his hand out-stretched, grabbed mine and shook it vigorously.

'The head porter told me to introduce myself to you, Sir. My name is Thomas and I'm new here, but if I am on duty when you are working, I'm at your service.'

Somewhat puzzled by his manner, I mumbled my thanks.

'I have just been discharged from Her Majesty's Guards. I have been in action with them, and we owe a great debt to you and your profession. It's an honour to know you.'

As he walked away, I stood bemused. I shrugged my shoulders and turned to get on with some work, only to find a group of grinning porters behind me.

'He's a queer chap,' I said, pointing to the retreating Thomas. 'He even addressed me as Sir. He's set you lot a good example. He knows a gentleman when he sees one.'

The resultant laughter puzzled me.

'What's funny?' I asked.

'We've just told him you're the head brain surgeon, and to treat you with great respect,' came the reply.

Alas Thomas' career as a porter was brief. During his short time at the hospital he weaved a web of fantasy about his past. The nearest he had been to having a military career was when he was a member of the Salvation Army, and all the tales about his background turned out to be untrue. Although the rest of the porters just ignored his stories, the hospital had to dispose of his services when he adopted the role of Dr Thomas to people living in the vicinity. It was later revealed that poor Thomas had spent some time in a mental institution before starting work in the Casualty Department.

But as Danny the porter remarked: 'I always said you have to be mad to work in this bloody place.'

* * *

'Are you busy, Walter?' Sister Sue asked as I finished changing the pillow cases on a trolley.

'No, what do you want, Sister?'

'Can you get me some ice cubes please?'

'Yes. How many do you want? There are a few in the kitchen fridge.'

'As many as you can get, a bagful at the very least.'

'Right, I'll go and scrounge some from the wards. Are they urgent?'

'I'd like them as soon as possible.'

She didn't say what size the bag had to be, and the only one I could find was a polythene one that someone had discarded in the kitchen that must have contained sandwiches, judging by the crumbs left at the bottom. I had to visit four wards to rob the fridges before collecting a reasonable amount of ice cubes, and it was some time later that I returned and found Sister Sue. I held the bag up before her eyes.

'Here you are, Sister. Where's the party? I have the ice, have you got the gin?'

'The party's this way, follow me.'

She led the way to a cubicle and lifted the curtain to reveal a young man in his early twenties lying on a trolley, covered by a white sheet.

'You will soon be alright now, Mr Morgan,' Sister said. 'We have our resident organ specialist to help you.' She turned to me. 'Carry on, Walter.'

My bewilderment must have shown on my face. Not wishing to appear a fool in front of the patient, I turned to Sister and whispered, 'What am I supposed to do?'

'Put the bag of ice cubes round his penis and get the swelling down.'

'His penis!'

'Yes, take a look at it.'

She pulled back the white sheet to reveal a massive organ. It was an unhealthy shade of red, and the blue veins stood out in relief as it stood so proud. I had no idea what its real size should have been, but it must have swelled to four or five times bigger than normal. My face must have changed to a deeper shade of red than the patient's penis.

'Can't he do it himself?' I whispered again.

'No, we want him on his back so we can check him. Stay with him, Walter, I'll send one of the nurses in when I have one free.' She turned and left the cubicle.

Wearing rubber gloves, I surrounded the huge stump with ice cubes, and I wondered what topic of conversation would interest the patient to take his mind off his unfortunate situation. I could hardly talk about the weather; to say that it had turned out nice again didn't seem quite appropriate. Perhaps he was interested in sport. But as I eyed the swollen organ I thought perhaps he indulged in a different kind of sport from the one I had in mind. So I restricted myself by asking him if the ice was helping to reduce the swelling, although I must admit his penis still looked as big as ever. Probably the poor fellow was as embarrassed as I was, because he didn't answer. As I kept building up the ice cubes round the penis, I noticed that they had melted to some degree, and I started speculating whether the hospital would run out of ice before any reduction in size was achieved.

It was all of twenty minutes later when the curtains parted and Sister returned with a staff nurse.

'Has it gone down yet?' she asked.

'Not at all,' I replied.

'You can take over now, Staff Nurse. Thank you, Walter, for your help.'

The staff nurse looked rather dubious as she stepped forward and surveyed the patient.

'What am I supposed to do?' she asked.

Sister gazed down at the still gigantic penis.

‘You could start by offering him free bed and breakfast,’ she replied.

* * *

Relations between the porters and patients were generally good. This was because the patients perhaps felt vulnerable in the midst of all the activity that was going on around them while they were waiting to see the doctor, or to receive treatment. They were always interested in the working conditions of the staff and all asked the same questions, and made the same remarks.

‘What time do you start work?’ Or ‘What time do you finish work?’

‘These trolleys are like those in the supermarkets, they have minds of their own.’

‘Oh, you are good people. How would we manage without you?’

During a National Health pay dispute, it always caused the staff great amusement when I was told by patients, “I hope you get your pay rise.” I usually replied that I was hoping to get two more noughts at the end of my monthly salary.

Very sick patients were escorted to the wards by a nurse, but the porters were often unaccompanied when taking patients on routine visits to clinics, and to the X-ray department. A patient’s condition could deteriorate very rapidly, and by alerting the staff the porters helped to avoid some serious situations. Unexpected cardiac arrests were not uncommon, and patients waiting to see the doctor were closely monitored after being checked by the nursing staff. On one occasion a man was found dead on his trolley, although he had been seen by a doctor just after his arrival.

The constant stream of vehicles in the ambulance bay,

with the ever-changing faces of the people inside them, kept the department permanently busy. Some people were beyond help on their arrival, and the doctor on duty would go into the vehicle to check the corpse before it was removed to the winter gardens. There was little comfort the staff could offer the weeping relatives who may have accompanied the ambulance, and it was not an easy journey when at times the sister on duty asked me to drive them home in my car.

The Grim Reaper swings his scythe without fear of favour, and it was always a sad moment when I actually helped push the glory wagon to the winter gardens, knowing that it contained someone I knew, sometimes a friend or an acquaintance. The staff of the hospital were themselves mortal, and some of the porters who had previously pushed the vehicle to the winter gardens also took their last ride in it.

Hospital porters working in the Casualty Department in my early days were unique individuals. Much maligned by some of the staff, they worked long shifts for poor wages, acted as security officers (often assaulted by violent patients) helped in the maintenance of the department at night and removed victims to the mortuary who had died in the most traumatic circumstances. Even now, through the corridor of time, I can still hear the voices of the staff in the Casualty Department shouting, "Porter ... PORTER".

Chapter 5

Accident and Emergency

Medicine is an inexact science

The Accident and Emergency Department stood on the opposite side of the road from the main hospital, and it was connected by an overhead bridge and an underground tunnel. Very few people referred to the department as the Accident and Emergency, despite the insistence of the consultant in charge. It was always casualty or "Cas".

To reach the department, patients and visitors had to turn into a small side street and follow the sign which read "Accidents Only", as it was the only accessible building in the area. On the outside wall near the main entrance, and set in the stonework, a huge pair of hands stood out in relief. Cradled between them was a small figure of a man, who appeared at first sight to be slipping through the extended fingers. But when viewed from a more acute angle, one got the impression that he was about to be thrown towards the public toilets at the end of the street.

Large "Keep Clear" notices marked the parking bays for the ambulances, which everyone seemed to disregard, much to the annoyance of the ambulance drivers. Arrows on the outside walls pointed the way to the main entrance through a battered door which had suffered from the kicks of numerous patients and rowdy drunks, who had found it easier to enter by using their feet instead of their hands.

Inside the building on the left-hand side was a large desk, on which rested the telephones, the record book and the casualty cards. The desk at that time was staffed during the day by female receptionists and at night by a solitary male clerk. There was a large waiting room on the right-hand side of the foyer, and it was furnished with chairs and small tables. These were a great improvement on the hard wooden forms that had constituted the original seating arrangements. Signs pointed the way to the fracture clinic, which consisted of two very small rooms – a gross exaggeration of the word "clinic". There was also an X-ray department boasting its own waiting room that could just about hold four patients, providing they were of normal size, and in the centre of this area stood the curtained cubicles to screen the incoming patients. Although they were hidden from passing eyes, their privacy was limited as every word uttered behind the drapes by the patients and staff could be overheard by any casual bystander. Serious emergency cases were rushed into the resuscitation room that stood just inside the ambulance bay containing the life support equipment, but it was very small and there was only room for one patient, which meant that any other emergencies had to be treated in the cubicles, and on occasions this created some problems.

For several years until the new Casualty Department opened, this was my weekend world. From early Saturday evening to Sunday morning, I was divorced from my normal professional life that took place the rest of the week. My whole concept of moral and social values changed as I came face to face with the dark side of humanity: the sick, the distressed, the violent, the victims of violence, and the endless stream of people suffering from some form of injury or illness.

A well known London theatre had a slogan during the last war which read "We Never Close", and Casualty Departments could also make the same claim. But within its walls was a theatre of a different kind, where life and death dramas were played out daily. No dramatist or writer of fiction could imagine the varied and bizarre situations that were enacted here, or even do justice to the characters that crowded this stage, and who took their bows before disappearing into the wings for ever. The knife edge between farce and tragedy, tears and laughter, was balanced on at this establishment for 24 hours a day, every day of the year. The doors of the Accident and Emergency Department were always open and the whole spectrum of human behaviour was laid bare before the people who worked there.

The popular image of beautiful nurses cooling the fevered brows of grateful patients, and of doctors performing miracles, dies a hard death in any casualty department. Hard work, unsocial hours and poor pay seems to be written into every hospital worker's contract. But rising above the stink of vomit, unwashed bodies, urine and other human waste matter, there was always a sense of compassion. The staff were not there to make any moral judgements on the patients they treated, only to offer help. Even when they were working under great pressure, they usually found time to utter a word of reassurance to a patient, or an expression of sympathy to a bereaved relative. These gestures did not come easily when the long hours of duty took their toll, and the sound of a telephone ringing could herald a new emergency. There is no glamour in the medical and nursing professions, but there is fulfilment in the lives of most of the staff who are engaged in this work. I was fortunate to be able to share it with them.

The staff of the department were constantly changing, and as each new intake arrived for training, I was forever forming new relationships. The permanent members of staff continued to demand discipline and vigorous study to promote excellence. But the newcomers were always puzzled by my appearance on the scene in my white coat, by my lack of authority, and my relationship with the porters, the receptionists and the nurses. The white coat usually earmarked me as a doctor, but when the mystery was solved, and they discovered that I could be very helpful just by doing my mundane work, the bonds were formed and a new cycle of acceptance had begun.

My Saturday work varied according to the sister who was on duty. Most evenings started with me taking over the consulting room and acting as the casualty officer's receptionist in the area used for receiving minor injuries. I called the patients from the waiting room for their consultation, and afterwards directed the walking cases to the X-ray department, the fracture clinic or the treatment room. I received many strange looks when I asked the ladies with leg and foot injuries if they would remove their tights before seeing the doctor. This was for him to examine the site of the injury, but on many occasions I had to restrain some patients from taking them off in the corridor where I was working, before I could direct them to a nearby room. One old lady started to struggle with her undies, to the embarrassment of the onlookers, so that the doctor could examine her in-growing toe-nail.

These duties lasted until 9 o'clock in the evening when the consulting rooms were closed down, and the night shift took over. I then reverted to my work as a porter-cum-errand boy and reception clerk. As the shifts changed, so did my name. It was Fred, Bill, John or whatever came to mind. But the porters solved the problem by referring to me as the Pox Doctor's Clerk, a title in keeping with their hospital humour.

The non-medical staff made a great contribution to the efficient running of the department. Included in this category were the clerks, cleaners and maintenance men. But the porters were in a special class of their own. Perhaps it was working closely with them and sharing their experience at first hand that made me so aware of their value to the Casualty Department and to the hospital. Their services were required everywhere during those early days. They had to relieve the telephonists and the male night receptionist, wrestle with the drunks, take the sick to the wards, remove the dead to the mortuary and act as errand boys carrying blood samples and X-ray plates to their required destinations. The mortuary visits did not appeal to some of the portering staff, and I was never compelled to do this duty, but there were times, owing to shortage of staff and pressure of work, when it was necessary, as it required two people for the task. After a time it became part of the routine, and after all, I was no use as a voluntary worker if I was not prepared to cover all aspects of the job.

In any accident and emergency department the staff come face to face with death throughout the year. People who had been involved in road traffic accidents [R.T.As.], people who had collapsed in the street and been brought in dead [B.I.Ds], people taking overdoses [O.Ds]. There were also victims of violence – murder or manslaughter – and suicides by hanging, wrist-slitting, setting themselves on fire, jumping from buildings, running in front of cars, inhaling poisonous gasses, electrocution and drowning. The ways to commit suicide were endless, and all the cases were subject to investigation by a coroner or a Home Office pathologist. One wondered if the people who destroyed themselves realised the trauma they left as a legacy for their friends and relatives.

To remove the remains we used the specially constructed trolley. This vehicle stood out of sight in the basement, outside a small room that was known as the porters' lodge, but in reality the place contained a few lockers, and a kettle for making tea. The glory wagon was constructed out of sheet metal, and basically it was a box on wheels with a lid that folded over the top to hide the occupant. When it was necessary to use it in the early evening, we took devious routes to the mortuary to avoid the mainstream of visiting relatives.

The mortuary was approached from a basement corridor,

through some double doors and across a courtyard to the building itself. The entrance was at the top of a ramp leading to the main door. At night and at weekends the porters had the keys to the place as the mortuary staff were not usually available during these periods. A journey to the Winter Gardens in the early hours of the morning, pushing our silent companion and lashed by snow and rain in the Winter, was an eerie task. The darkness of the courtyard enveloped us as we crossed it, and I always had a feeling of deep depression that stayed with me, along with the sickly sweet smell of death that lingered in the atmosphere of the Winter Gardens.

On some Sunday evenings, when we had to take a corpse to the Winter Gardens, we would discover Reg the mortician busy laying out the bodies on the stone tables and, with the tools of his trade, preparing them for examination by the pathologist on the following Monday morning. This procedure helped to save time during very busy periods, and Reg always seemed to enjoy his work. He would on occasions invite us to share a pot of tea with him, but I always declined with thanks, as it was not exactly the right atmosphere to enjoy a cup, with all those naked bodies in the background.

* * *

The duties of the sister, or the male charge nurse, who were in charge of the nursing staff in the Casualty Department were quite varied. Apart from their nursing duties, they had to liaise with the Social Services, the Police, the Ambulance Service, and many other organisations. They had to reassure patients, comfort distressed relatives, and explain to the parents of little Willie, without breaking any code of ethics, that the doctors were very busy looking after the victim of a road traffic accident; that their son would not die from the effects of a cut finger, and that the very serious cases must get priority treatment.

As time passed many nursing sisters made fleeting appearances on the scene, but the pressures involved took their toll. The unsocial hours affected their marriages, and the stress caused nervous breakdowns, and even an inclination towards drink. Some just faded away into oblivion whilst others will always remain in my memory.

Some of the names that the porters used to describe the nursing staff were very improper, and quite unjustified. But I thought one name was well chosen for one sister at that time. They called her the Iron Maiden. She was in her early forties with short blonde hair that was cut in a schoolboy fashion. She was very upright in stature and walked with a grace that was rare. She never seemed to hurry, yet all her movements seemed to have a set purpose related to her work. There was an air of calmness about her, and this air always had a reassuring effect on the patients. She rarely smiled, which was a pity, for when she did the solemnity of her features took on a warm glow. She never wasted words on idle social chatter, and when she did speak it was to give directions to her staff. Her aloofness acted as a barrier, and she seemed to be a lonely figure, guarding her private thoughts and perhaps some secret sorrow.

The Iron Maiden demanded the highest standards of work from her staff, and accepted no excuses from the trained members who failed to conform; but she would go to great lengths to help the student nurses. Her mode of address was always formal, and she expected the same formalities in return. Many young doctors made the mistake of being too familiar, but they soon realised their folly, and confined their relationship to a working one. Most of the staff disliked her, but everyone respected her for the efficiency and drive she brought to the department when she was on duty. She knew what to do in any emergency, and made sure her staff did too.

Although the Iron Maiden was hard in her attitudes to the people under her control, she was even harder on herself. When the department was working under pressure, she would ensure that her staff had their breaks, but never took one herself. She always set an example to the rest of the department, and if she took any staff member aside to criticise their work, the criticism was usually merited.

I also discovered another thing about the Iron Maiden. She did not like voluntary workers.

When she was on duty and I appeared on the scene, she completely ignored me. There was no greeting for me, and as far as she was concerned I did not exist. All her instructions were addressed to the porters, and if they were not at hand she would wait until one appeared. I felt quite isolated. There were other areas, however, that she did not control, so I did work on odd jobs in the fracture clinic, the X-ray department and on the reception desk. The porters did show some resentment at the loss of an extra pair of hands during their busy periods, but could do nothing to alter the situation. With hindsight, I can look back and realise the reluctance of the Iron Maiden to accept a part-time amateur in her team. She expected the highest professional conduct from everyone, and therefore an outsider like me just did not fit in.

Perhaps it was my initial dislike of her that made me stay when she was on duty. I had been accepted over the years, and built up a very good relationship with the rest of the staff, who welcomed my help. After all, I was working there with the consent of the management, so I dug me heels in and stayed.

It was late one Saturday night when the breakthrough occurred. It was a strange night, and for the hospital a very peaceful one. There were more staff on duty than patients waiting to be treated, and there seemed to be an atmosphere of impending doom prevailing in the department. I was sitting with Ron, the night clerk, at the reception desk, well out of the way of the Iron Maiden. I yawned and turned to him.

'It's quiet tonight, Ron.'

'Too bloody quiet. I don't like it.'

'There must be a good show on television.'

'You should ask my wife. She watches everything on the box. According to her, T.V. is better than having sex.'

It was then that the radio transmitter that was on link with the ambulance control burst into life, along with the strident ring of one of the telephones on the desk. Ron indicated to me to answer the phone while he acknowledged the radio call.

'Accident and Emergency.'

'This is Ambulance Control. Is Sister there?'

There was no need to ask, as the Iron Maiden was standing by my side. She had obviously been alerted by the loud noise on the radio, and Ron shouting down the microphone. I passed the handset to her, and thought it better to make my exit, as she would not want me around. I wandered off along the corridor and busied myself stripping some used beds and changing the blankets. As I worked, I could hear the voice of the Iron Maiden in the distance issuing orders, and then I saw her approaching, accompanied by Milly the staff nurse, who came up to me.

'Where are all the porters, Walter?'

'There are only five on duty tonight, Staff. At this time they'll be relieving on the telephone exchange on the wards, and perhaps in the theatres.'

'There's been a multiple pile up on the motorway with some fatalities. We're not sure of the number, but so far there are at least six patients on the way. Get some trolleys ready in the ambulance bay, I'll round up the rest of the porters and get them down here.'

'Right, Staff.'

The Iron Maiden gave me a fleeting glance, but she added nothing to the Staff Nurse's instructions and turned away. I had the trolleys all lined up before the other porters arrived on the scene, but there were still not enough. Nine people were injured in the crash, four seriously, and two dead bodies still trapped in the wreckage had yet to be released. It was a night of unceasing effort for a depleted staff. I helped undress some of the patients, there were blood samples to be matched, numerous visits to the X-ray department to be made, patients to be taken to the wards and of course all the paperwork. Poor Ron on the reception desk was crying out for my help at the same time as the porters were calling for me. Another badly-injured man expired but it was some time before we could make a journey to the Winter Gardens with his remains. It was a bloody night with no relief for the staff apart from the large teapot that I constantly kept refilled in one of the side rooms.

The Saturday night and Sunday morning drunks now filled the waiting room and Ron was being badly abused by them for keeping them waiting; but fortunately the police who had now arrived on the scene came to his aid and restored some order. It was impossible to reason with the drunks, who were suffering mostly from some minor injury, usually self-inflicted, and you could not describe the trauma to them that existed behind the scenes. Quite a number of patients expected a rotation procedure, like a cinema queue, and never made allowances for serious cases.

The early morning sun was just breaking through the clouds as the last of the crash victims was trundled into a ward, and the nursing staff was clearing away some of the debris from the treatment rooms. I had finished helping the porters mop up the blood on a cubicle floor. Another night was over, and I took off my white doctor's coat, now badly stained, and went into the staff room to claim my own clothes. It was going home time. It had been a sad night, and it was going to be an even sadder day for the relatives and friends of the victims. I realised how weary I was, and the mental image of a pot of coffee and a bed inspired me to move my leaden legs along the corridor. As I passed the half-open door of Sister's office, I wondered if the Iron Maiden felt as I did. I had caught glimpses of her over the last few hours. She had not spoken, but there had been no orders for me to stop my activities. I had reacted in my own way to the incident as the situation developed. I was almost at the door when a voice addressed me from behind.

'Mr Cockshaw.'

I turned round slowly; my weary limbs needed coaxing into action. The Iron Maiden was standing outside her office, her head held high.

'Yes, Sister?'

'Thank you for your help.'

She turned round and hurried along the corridor to the treatment cubicles. As I stood awhile, her voice came echoing back.

'... Nurse, I thought I told you to put those splints away, I don't want them lying around ...'

I went in search of my car, now walking on air.

* * *

It was always possible to tell the seasons of the year in the Casualty Department. Autumn and Winter brought in the footballers and hockey players, whereas Spring heralded the beginning of the fly-fishing season, when a large number of anglers managed to sink hooks into every conceivable parts of their bodies – a sort of poetic justice, which I am sure would have delighted the fish. In Summer the victims of demon bowlers and aspiring batsmen from the local cricket fields came nursing their injuries, some accompanied by their wives or girlfriends who showed them little sympathy, and constantly harangued them to give up the silly game.

During this period the school children had their long holidays, and it was amazing how many of them managed to fall out of trees, get knocked off their bicycles, chew poisonous berries, get bitten by dogs, break their bones. The list of injuries were endless. Some were allied to whatever sporting event was appearing on their television screens, as the kids emulated their heroes playing in the World Cup matches, Test Matches and the Olympics.

All through the year there were patients of both sexes who were admitted at a steady rate; these were the would-be suicides, most of whom made this traumatic gesture as a cry for help rather than a serious attempt to kill themselves. The doctors could only try to repair the damage that they had inflicted on themselves, and then pass them on to someone who could give them psychiatric help, as the Casualty Department was not an ideal place for counselling. The time came when I ceased to be shocked, surprised or even revolted by what I saw or heard. I accepted the prostitutes, the sexual deviants, the alcoholics, the violent and the victims of violence as being the normal sequence of events, and I no longer tried to classify people into groups by their lifestyle. The department was a melting pot for the whole of humanity, and it could not be changed, only accepted.

Among the many patients to pass through the doors were individuals suffering from mental disorders. Some would be found wandering in the city streets, and the police or the ambulance men would bring them to the hospital. Others would be reported by anxious neighbours or relatives who had become alarmed at their irrational behaviour. Before these patients could be detained and removed to a mental hospital, they had to be examined by a psychiatrist and a representative from the Social Services, and sectioned under the Mental Health Act. There was usually a delay before the on-duty officers could be contacted, and as these patients could not be left on their own, it was necessary for someone to sit with them. So when the staff were busy, I was usually given the task. Over the years I spent many hours listening to the out-pourings of these unfortunate people.

The job was not without its hazards however, as some patients could be quite violent, and one had to be careful when conversing with them.

Peter was one such person. He was a young man in his early twenties, and as I sat with him, he started telling me about the book he had written that contained all the secrets of the universe. To keep him pacified I showed great interest in it, and expressed a desire to read it.

'Why do you want to read it?' he asked.

'So I can learn about life,' I replied.

I must have given him the wrong answer. He rose casually from the wooden chair he was sitting on, and in a flash he picked it up, swung it round and attempted to batter my skull with it. Fortunately, I stepped aside and received the blow on my shoulder. Two of the porters who were in the vicinity came rushing across and helped me to restrain him before he could repeat his efforts. As we struggled he started screaming:

'You son of Satan. You want to steal my holy secrets!'

The noise echoed along the corridor, and Sister, along with several members of the staff, came dashing on the scene.

'What the hell is going on?' she demanded.

'It's alright, Sister,' said one of the porters. 'Mr Cockshaw has just discovered who his father is.'

It was obvious that my popularity had reached a low ebb

with Peter, and it was decided that some feminine company would have a soothing effect on him. So he was taken to a side room and a pretty young nurse was detailed to stay with him. He also accepted a cup of tea with profound thanks, which he promptly poured into the nurse's lap as she sat next to him. After that, two porters took over the duty of watching him, as Sister decided that one bruised shoulder and a change of knickers was enough trouble for one night.

* * *

From simple beginnings some situations can become highly embarrassing. A patient by the name of Ann was discovered in a shop doorway by the police, who had been alerted by a passer-by. They found Ann trying to strangle herself by looping a length of cord round her neck and pulling it tight with both hands. She was brought into Casualty by an ambulance for her own safety, as the red weals round her neck were grim evidence of her intentions. It was obvious that she could not be left alone as she waited for the psychiatrist, so a staff nurse was detailed to sit with her in a prominent position in the corridor. It was while I was changing some blankets on the trolleys that Ann and her escort passed me and entered the ladies' toilet at the end of the corridor. Then things started to happen. A minute or two later the nurse's face appeared round the door of the loo, and a voice that contained a note of panic echoed along the corridor.

'Walter! Walter! Give me a hand!'

I left what I was doing and hurried towards her.

'What's the matter?' I enquired.

'Ann has locked herself in the lavatory, she's a suicidal case and I'm supposed to be looking after her. If she harms herself I'll get the blame.' She seemed very close to tears.

'Don't worry, love, I'm an expert at rescuing old ladies from lavatories. Is she alone in there?'

'Yes.'

Ladies' lavatories were a no-go area for me, but the nurse was obviously upset; and as there was no one else around, some reassurance on my part might help to ease the situation. (I did get quite familiar with this particular block of toilets later on, when I helped to rescue other female patients who were suffering from an excess of alcohol.)

I followed the nurse inside and there were three toilets in line. Two of them had their doors open, but the one nearest the wall was closed. I tried to put it open but it was locked from the inside. The nurse knocked on the door and in a quiet voice implored Ann to unlock it, but there was no reply, and her anxiety increased. Time passed and the situation was getting more serious. It was then I noticed the radiator on the side of the wall. I grabbed the top of the wooden partition above the toilet door, put my foot on the radiator top and heaved myself up. By doing so I could just get my body through the gap between the top of the door and the ceiling, and by leaning over inside I could just release the catch that held the door. It swung open.

Ann was on the floor, this time with a belt round her neck, and she was tugging it with both her hands. It was with some difficulty that we managed to relieve her of it, but she seemed no worse off for her ordeal. The nurse escorted her back along the corridor with a sigh of relief, thankful that no further harm had come to her charge.

It was a strange thing that when I got involved in an incident it had no completion but went on and on like some soap opera with the usual commercial breaks in between. It was like this with Ann. I was just having my commercial break in the kitchen with a cup of tea when I heard the nurse's voice calling me once again.

'Walter! Walter! Give me a hand.'

I put my teacup down reluctantly and looked round the door. Just along the corridor the nurse was wrestling with Ann. The nurse wasn't a very big girl and she was losing out in the power struggle. With an upsurge of energy, Ann wrenched herself free, pushed the nurse against the wall and streaked away along the corridor towards the ladies' toilets again. The nurse, obviously now quite shaken, picked herself up off the floor, and waving to me to join her, followed hard on Ann's heels. I took another sip of my tea, breathed a sigh, and got ready to do my Tarzan act again. I wandered slowly down to the ladies' loo. The nurse stood waiting with a worried expression on her face.

'She's locked herself in again, Walter.'

'Don't worry, I'll get her out.'

'Oh, Thanks.'

I went inside and once again the door of the cubicle nearest the wall was closed, while the other two were open. It was locked from the inside so I didn't hesitate. I heaved myself up, swung my body through the gap at the top and stretched my hand downwards towards the catch. I soon realised that all was not well. A pair of startled eyes gazed up at me, and a mouth opened in terror. There was a woman inside, but it wasn't Ann.

Even now, many years later, I have visions of an uplifted skirt, white thighs, pink knickers and rumpled tights every time I see a sign marked "Ladies". I have no idea how long we both stared at each other, but I do remember saying 'I beg your pardon' before I dropped to the floor. Then she started to scream. Well, it wasn't so much a scream but more like a siren. It rose from a wail to a penetrating frequency which echoed down the corridors to the outside yard. I was told later by Ken the porter that it stopped everyone in their tracks. They thought that the Last Trumpet had sounded, or that a nuclear war had started. How she managed to maintain that scream for so long I just don't know, but I hope she donates her lungs to medical science when she passes on as they must be unique.

The ladies' toilet was suddenly full of jabbering people milling round and asking questions without getting any answers. The nurse was trying to explain to Sister, who wasn't listening anyway. She was demanding to know why so many men were in the ladies' loo, as the porters and doctors were helping to swell the crowd. It was sheer chaos, with everyone talking at the same time, while the lady who had now emerged from her cubicle made helpless gestures in my direction, pinpointing me as the cause of all the trouble. The melee would have gone on much longer had not a female voice shouted, 'Do you mind getting out of here, I want to have a piss.'

It was one of our regular patients, old Nellie. The staff usually groaned when she came in to tell them all about her troubles, but for once I was glad to see her. She broke up the gathering, and the crowd started to disperse.

With all the consternation, I think I was the only one to remember that Ann was still missing. I discovered her in the broom cupboard that was in an alcove in the toilet. As it was only two foot square she couldn't sit down, and there was no item in there that she could strangle herself with. It was a great relief, and the cause of all the trouble was lead away once again.

The ensuing enquiry took place in Sister's office, with the lady from the loo being pacified with a cup of tea and an apology. After hearing my explanation, she seemed satisfied and agreed not to write to her MP and the Minister of Health. But even so, when she left the office I was convinced she still regarded me as a sex maniac by the way she scuttled past me and dashed out the door. I was also advised by a stern-faced

Sister to be careful about entering ladies' lavatories, and I nodded in agreement. But I could hear her laughter as I left her office.

* * *

While death was always close at hand in the Casualty Department, there were times when life renewed itself with the birth of a baby. Although the hospital had its own maternity unit, which was separate from the main building, very often expectant mothers were rushed in by mistake, usually by their worried husbands, and these patients were frequently so close to giving birth that it was not possible to transfer them in time to the maternity unit. Many of the young nurses were quite thrilled when this happened, but the more experienced ones were more cautious, knowing the dangers that were involved.

Sadly, some of the expectant mothers were young teenage girls still at school. They complained to their parents of severe abdominal pains and the parents, ignorant of their daughter's real condition, had by-passed their own doctors, as their surgeries had shut, to rush their daughters to Casualty. It was quite a shock for them to be told that they were going to be grandparents. The ages of the young mothers varied, but among the youngest was a girl of 13. It was hard at that early stage to determine the parents' feelings towards their daughters. The initial reaction in some cases was a sense of shame at the social stigma of having an illegitimate baby in the family; and some showed their anger towards their daughters. Time would help them come to terms with the situation, as both the new mothers and babies would need all the love, care and support their families could give.

Passing through the reception area one Saturday night,

Len the receptionist gave me a wave and beckoned me over to the desk.

'Get me a wheelchair, Walter, and take this young lady down to the cubicles.'

The patient concerned was a young girl aged about eighteen, rather plump, but nevertheless very pretty. She seemed to be in great pain, and she was making little moaning noises. There was an older woman with her who identified herself as her aunt. She was a very dominant lady, and as I returned with a wheelchair she was telling Len that her niece, who was a student at the local university, was staying with her, and was giving the poor man a diagnosis of the patient's condition.

'The poor girl must be suffering from appendicitis. I should know, I had the same pains before I had my appendix out. She should see a doctor immediately.'

Len had heard it all before, and he was completely immune to people's opinions.

'You must tell the doctor, madam. Follow that gentleman, he'll show you where to go.'

I pushed the girl along to the treatment cubicles, and luckily found the Sister in charge. 'What's wrong with this patient?' she asked.

Before I could answer, the girl's aunt broke in.

'She's got appendicitis. I want you to get her examined by a doctor at once.'

Sister's face hardened. She was not used to people telling her what to do. She called over Tracey, the staff nurse.

'Find a cubicle for this young lady, and help her get undressed. And do the preliminary observations.' She turned to the aunt, 'Would you stay in the waiting room, please.'

'But I want to stay with her.'

'We understand your concern, but we have no room for relatives in the cubicles. Apart from being too small, it does obstruct our staff. We'll keep you informed.' She turned away and auntie, somewhat red-faced, made her way back to the waiting room.

I wheeled the patient into a cubicle. She was still evidently in great pain, and the moaning grew louder. I helped Tracey to pick her up and put her on the bed. The girl cried out as we lifted her.

'Did the aunt say what was wrong with her?' Tracey asked.

'She says the girl has got appendicitis.'

Tracey placed her hands on the girl's stomach and pressed lightly.

'Bloody hell, Walter. Get the doctor and Sister. Her appendix is moving.'

The aunt's natural concern for the welfare of her niece was reflected in the way she expended her energy pacing up and down the corridor. She was extremely worried, but it was a great pity that her attitude towards the staff was so off-hand and abusive. She proved to be a great nuisance with her constant demands for information about her niece's appendicitis, and poor Len on the reception desk was on the receiving end of her complaints. After about thirty minutes of waiting she really lost her temper.

'I want to see my niece,' she went on, banging on the counter with her fist. 'I want to know what's happening to her.'

Len rose wearily from his desk for about the fifth time.

'Alright, Madam, I'll go and enquire again for you.' He turned and made the long walk down to the cubicles, leaving me in charge. He wasn't gone very long, and when he returned he had that poker-faced look on his face that usually heralded some profound statement.

'Well?' demanded the aunt. 'Is there any news?'

'Yes.'

'Are they going to remove my niece's appendix?'

'They've removed it.'

'Removed it already?'

'If you listen carefully,' Len went on, 'you will hear it crying.'

Above the noise of the distant traffic, and the hum of human activity, the sound of a baby crying could be heard from along the corridor as a new pair of lungs were exercised for the first time.

* * *

If the whole gamut of life and death can start and finish in the Casualty Department, then the intermediate stages of human relationships cannot be ignored. Marriage is a part of such a relationship.

Before weddings, then as now, many young couples had parties to celebrate their forthcoming nuptials, and these took the form of hen parties for the prospective brides, and stag parties for the bridegrooms. But what should be happy affairs often get out of hand through a surfeit of intoxicating beverages and horseplay, sometimes culminating in a visit to the Casualty Department.

Initiation ceremonies date back to the dark ages, and although they are still used for some secret societies and closed groups, they are not usually associated with people working at factory floor level. But it was the custom in one local engineering factory to launch the prospective bridegroom into the sea of matrimony in their own particular way. On the Friday lunchtime before the wedding, they would handcuff the poor unsuspecting victim to a convenient lamp-post or pole, partly strip him, and put a poster round his neck to advertise his coming nuptials. One such ceremony went wrong when someone lowered the victim's trousers and painted his penis. It was twelve hours later when the poor prospective groom found the courage to visit the Casualty Department to have the paint removed. He was in great pain and red with embarrassment. Because he was getting married in eleven hours' time, he was anxious to change the colour of his penis from a deep green to a more natural shade before his future wife saw it.

'If we can't remove the paint,' said Sister, 'let's hope that she's colour blind.'

Another incident involved a patient called Frank, who had invited his friends to a stag party to mourn the passing of his final days as a bachelor. It was about two o'clock in the morning when he was carried into the waiting room of the Casualty Department, leaving a trail of blood on the floor, much to the annoyance of the night cleaners who had just finished mopping. Frank was bent double and moaning with pain. With the help of his friends, I managed to get him into a wheelchair. The smell of alcohol permeated the atmosphere, and Frank's companions seemed to regard his plight as a huge joke.

'Go and book him in and stay in the waiting room,' I said, as I knew the staff would not want half a dozen of his drunken friends in the treatment area. I wheeled him round to the cubicles, and helped Sister and a staff nurse get him onto a trolley. The front of Frank's trousers was covered in blood, and then he started being sick, much to the annoyance of Sister, who had been trying to question him about his injury and getting no answers.

'What's happened to him?' she directed the question to me.

'I don't know. He was brought in by his friends. They are in the waiting room, almost as drunk as he is. I told them to stay there.'

'See if you can find out for me, Walter. I'll see them later. I don't want those drunken idiots round here, we have enough already.'

It took me longer to get the story from his friends than anticipated, as there were six drunken voices all talking at once, each trying to give me a version of the incident. I returned to Sister, who now had the doctor in attendance.

'Well?' she enquired. 'What happened?'

'He's getting married in two days' time.'

'He'll be lucky,' she said. 'Go on.'

'...he's been having a stag party...'

'I didn't think he'd been to a bible class.'

'Well, on his way home, he saw a flag pole outside a garage ...'

'So ...'

'His friends dared him to climb up to the top and steal the flag.'

'And did he?'

'Oh yes.'

'What's that got to do with his injury?'

'Well, he got the flag and slid down the pole ...'

'Yes?'

'... and forgot about the hook at the bottom that secures the rope ...'

'So ...'

'... he tore his testicles on it.'

Sister looked at me and paused. 'It sounds like a lot of balls to me,' she said.

I have found from experience that one's friends, always with the best intentions, love to spread bad news, and Frank's colleagues were no exception. His future bride, who had retired to her bed after her own drunken hen party, was aroused and given an embellished account of the incident, and she duly arrived at the hospital accompanied by her mother, suffering from a bout of hysterics and an overdose of vodka. She cheered up a little when she discovered that Frank was still alive, but then dissolved into tears when she was told the details of his injury. Her interview with the doctor did nothing to reassure her.

'Does that mean that he ... that we ... can't ...'

'I'm afraid so,' came the reply.

'But we were going to get married on Saturday.' The tears were streaming down her face.

'Well, you may be able to get married, but you will have to postpone the honeymoon.'

When I left the department some time later the girl was weeping in the corner of the waiting room, being comforted by her mother, while on the other side, Frank's friends raised their voices in song as they waited for a taxi to take them home.

> *'Frank's getting married in the morning. Ding-dong the wedding bells will chime. He's been having fun and frolics. But he's slid and tore his bollocks. But we'll get him to the church on time.'*

* * *

'Take some good deep breaths,' said the staff nurse.

The patient lay on his side, and I held his arms behind him to restrain him from pulling the tube that was down his throat.

'I've nearly finished,' she went on. 'I hope you don't take another overdose, it doesn't solve any of your domestic problems, it only makes matters worse.'

Stomach wash-outs were part of the routine in the Casualty Department, and Ernie had taken a bottle of aspirin because of some family problem. After he had taken them, however, he'd had second thoughts about dying, which is not unusual in overdose patients, so he rang for an ambulance and was now undergoing gastric lavage.

We were in the resuscitation room, a small area with just enough room for the trolley that Ernie lay on. The room was equipped with the life support system usually reserved for more serious cases, such as people suffering from heart attacks or multiple injuries. It was inadequate for the needs of such a busy department, and already plans were being formulated to build an entirely new Accident and Emergency complex. But that was in the future, so in the meantime it was convenient for the staff to use the room for stomach wash-outs, as it was away from the busy treatment area, and caused less distress to the patients.

The staff nurse and I had been discussing what Ernie had been eating that day. It was a sort of guessing game that we played as we watched the remains of his meals, mixed with the undissolved tablets and traces of blood that had been regurgitated into a bucket by the side of the trolley, via a tube that was down his throat. We had almost finished when Sister came in.

'Have you nearly finished, Staff Nurse?' she asked. 'We have a cardiac arrest patient on the way. We shall need this room.'

'Right, Sister we'll clear up right away.' She turned to Ernie. 'I'm taking the tube out of your throat. Now, give a little cough.'

Ernie duly obliged, and I wheeled him into the corridor and helped the staff nurse clean the room. We finished just in time, as the ambulance, still with its blue lamp flashing, pulled into the bay. The unconscious patient was a man of about sixty years of age who had collapsed in the street. The doctors were already working on him as Sister and I started to undress him, beginning at the bottom. The procedure was automatic with me: shoes, socks and trousers, while Sister managed the top half. No words were spoken, and already the E.C.G. machine was linked up by the staff. Now it was up to the professionals, all I could do was watch.

The patient was surrounded by white-clad figures, and from my vantage point it was hard to see what was happening. There was a brief picture of a doctor giving cardiac massage, and then everyone stood back when the defibulator was used to send electrical impulses to the patient's heart. The combined efforts started again, and then a male voice said above the hum of activity: 'Bloody hell, he's gone again.' For another fifteen minutes the team worked with a cycle of successes and failures, but it was all in vain, and with a shrug the leader turned away. 'You win some, you lose some. We did our best,' was his final remark.

I was to witness the same scene but with different actors a great many times in the future. Now another phase of hospital procedure took over. As the patient had died in the street, he had to be officially identified by a member of his family, or someone who knew him.

'We shall need the body putting in the viewing room,' Sister remarked to Danny the porter. 'The police have gone to notify his relatives. Will you arrange it?'

'Leave it to me, Sister.'

The viewing room was a small extension of the mortuary. It was furnished with dark curtains, and the lights were controlled by dimmer switches to help avoid the stress that some relatives suffered during identification. There was a long table in the centre of the room for the body to be laid out on and a white sheet was placed over the corpse with the top turned down just to reveal the face. It was always an emotional task, and in the absence of the mortuary staff at night and at weekends, the porters always undertook the duty of making the deceased presentable for the relatives to view. I helped Danny, and we returned to Casualty to find Sister waiting.

'Have you taken the body down yet, Danny?'

'Yes, Sister, we've just done it.'

'I forgot to give you his dentures. Could you slip down and put them in, he'll look better when his family come to identify him.'

'I'd better do it now,' Danny replied and taking the denture box from Sister, he disappeared down the stairs again, leaving me to carry on with stripping the trolleys that had been used by the patients in our absence, and renewing the blankets. As I worked I noticed an ambulance pull into the bay, and Michael the driver came in whistling. He stopped when he saw me.

'Is Sister about?' he asked.

'She's in her office.'

'Oh well, give her these. I'm in a hurry.'

He pushed a tissue wrapped bundle in my hand. I examined it with some suspicion. The contents felt hard as my fingers probed the wrapping.

'What are these?'

'Dentures.'

'Dentures? Why do we want them?'

'Tell Sister that they belong to the cardiac patient who died. I took them out of his mouth on the way here in the ambulance when I was trying to resuscitate him, and I forgot them in the emergency.'

'I think you must be mistaken. Danny's just taken some dentures down to the mortuary to fit them in his mouth.'

'I assure you they are. I took them out myself.'

'You'd better come and have a word with Sister.'

We found her in her office having a quiet cup of tea and smoking a cigarette, which rather surprised me, as she always lectured the patients about the evils of smoking. Michael explained the reason for his visit.

'Oh my God!' she exclaimed. 'Let's get hold of Danny quick before the relatives arrive to identify the body.'

She grabbed the dentures out of my hand, and leaving her tea and her cigarette burning in an ashtray, she dashed out of the room and confronted Danny who was just stepping out of the lift.

'Have you fitted those dentures in yet, Danny?' she asked, her voice showed concern.

'I certainly have,' he gasped. 'And what a bloody job I had getting them in his mouth. The poor bugger's grinning like a Cheshire cat, as though he's glad to be dead.'

'Well, you had better go and take the grin off his face, they're the wrong ones. Go and swap them for these.'

Sister gently placed the tissue-wrapped package into the bewildered porter's hand, and retreated to her office and her cup of tea, leaving Danny to make his third visit to the mortuary.

Procedures laid down by the hospital authorities to safeguard patients' property and effects are usually strictly adhered to, but there are times in emergency situations when the patient's life may be at stake, and the time is so limited that they can be overlooked. Putting a name on a box of dentures can be of low priority for staff dealing with a cardiac arrest.

But fate took a hand in this sequence of events. The afternoon shift changed over to the night shift, and for a time the incident was forgotten. That is, until I took some X-rays to one of the wards. I walked quietly to the nurse's station where a solitary figure in white sat at her desk, illuminated by an angle-poise lamp. She looked up at my approach.

‘I’ve brought you your X-rays, Staff,’ I whispered so I didn’t wake up the patients.

‘Oh, thanks.’

It was then that the peace and quiet of the ward was shattered by a voice bellowing out of the darkness from a bed opposite the staff nurse’s desk.

‘That’s him. That’s him. He knows where they are.’

‘Shush, Mr Smith, you’ll wake the whole ward.’

But Mr Smith wouldn’t be shushed and continued to bellow.

‘He knows where they are, he knows.’

I had no idea what I was supposed to know. ‘What was that all about?’ I asked the nurse when she came back to her desk.

He’s a patient from Casualty who was admitted tonight.’

‘What’s wrong with him?’

‘He’s an overdose. He’s lost his false teeth somewhere, and he won’t go to sleep until we’ve found them. He’s driving me up the wall.’

The words overdose and false teeth set my brain working overtime. Perhaps I could solve the mystery of Mr Smith’s missing molars.

‘Can I take a look at the patient, Staff?’

‘Anything to keep him quiet.’

She drew the curtains around the bed and switched on the light. Blinking up at me was Ernie, the patient we had been treating before the cardiac arrest victim had been rushed into the resuscitation room. Now all was revealed. It was Ernie’s dentures that Danny the porter had been trying to fit into the mouth of the deceased man. His molars must still have been in Casualty.

‘Just relax, Mr Smith. We have your teeth in Casualty. I’ll go and get them for you.’

The nurse put out the light, and as we moved out of earshot I gave her an abbreviated version of what had happened, mentioning the fact that the teeth had been mixed up and used by another patient, though I thought it best not to tell that he was dead at the time.

'Thank Heaven you've found them,' she said. 'He's been on about his bloody choppers since he arrived in the ward.'

Life is never as simple as one imagines, and the saga of Ernie's false teeth was still to continue. On my return to Casualty, the place was still as busy as ever. There were two drunks fighting in the waiting room, a young girl was being sick in the corridor, and a crowd of youths were having a race in hospital wheelchairs in the ambulance bay. It was hardly the ideal time to enquire about Ernie's false teeth, but when order was restored I managed to catch up with Sister.

'I'm looking for some dentures, Sister.'

'Well, you can't have mine.'

I hurriedly explained the situation to her as the turmoil started again in the waiting room.

'I wonder if the previous shift had handed over any dentures to you before they went off duty?'

She paused for a second.

'I did give a box of dentures to the nurse on the Casualty Ward to put in the lost property cupboard, as no one seemed to know who they belonged to. Have a word with her... Don't let her be sick on the floor again... Get a vomit bowl...' She left me standing in the corridor.

The Casualty Ward was at the far end of the corridor, and it was divided into two sections, one for men and the other for women. Each section had six available beds, and these were generally used for patients who were admitted for overnight observation. The Nurse in charge sat in a central position so she could observe both sections. She sat writing at her desk as I entered.

'The teapot's empty,' she said without looking up.

'I don't want any tea, I'm looking for some dentures.'

'Well you can't have mine.' That joke again.

'Did Sister give you a denture box when she came on duty tonight?'

'I wonder what's on the menu for supper tonight ... yes, she did.'

'Never mind supper, can I have the dentures? They belong to a patient on a ward, and he can't get to sleep because he's worried about them.'

'I suppose it's chips with everything again ... I put them with the others.'

'Others? What others?'

'The others in the cupboard.'

She removed a key from her desk drawer, moved over to the corner of the room to a small cupboard and unlocked the door. I followed her. 'Take you pick,' she said gesturing to the contents inside. There on the centre shelf stood two rows of denture boxes. I counted up to nine at the front, and there were others behind. One of them must have contained Ernie's missing teeth, but which one? I had visions of spending the night trying to fit them in his mouth until I found the right ones. I knew exactly how the Prince felt before he found Cinderella, it must have been total despair. But she was at least a beautiful girl, and by no stretch of the imagination could you call Ernie beautiful. Even the Ugly Sisters would have looked glamorous compared to him. I turned to the Nurse.

'Where the hell did you get this lot from, a dentist's clearance sale?'

'Oh, the toilets.'

'The toilets?'

'Yes some of the drunks go in there to be sick, they take their false teeth out, put them on the window ledge and forget them. They wake up next morning and have no idea what's happened to them. The cleaners hand them in at the reception desk, so we keep them in here to be claimed. I think a lot of people are too ashamed to call in for them. It's about time we had a clear-out.'

'Don't have a clear-out before I've rescued Ernie's choppers.' This had now turned into a holy crusade for me.

The nurse reached forward to touch the boxes.

'Don't touch!' I yelled, forgetting that there were patients asleep in the ward.

'There's no need to shout. It's not my fault.'

'I'm sorry, but I must get the right set. Can you remember where you put them on the shelf?'

She leaned forward and paused. 'It could be that box,' she said, and touched one on the left hand side of the front row. 'But on the other hand, it could be this one.' She lifted up the box on the right.

I looked in both boxes. They both contained top and bottom sets. It was a start, so I took them both, and after sterilising them and washing them under the tap, I decided to take a chance that one of the sets must belong to Ernie. I made my way back to the ward where the same staff nurse greeted me.

'Have you found them?'

'I think so. Is Mr Smith still awake?'

'Yes, I am,' a voice answered from the shadows.

'Do you want the light on?' the nurse enquired.

'No, don't bother.'

I didn't want Ernie to realise my desperation. It was better for me to do the fitting in the dark. Keeping my fingers crossed I moved over to his bed and handed him the first set of dentures. He took the upper one and tried it in his mouth.

'These bloody teeth are not mine!' he yelled.

'I'm sorry, I must have given you the wrong ones, it's dark in here. Try these.' And as I handed him the other set I said a silent prayer.

There was a clinking of jaws, and a grunt from the darkness. 'These are mine,' said Ernie, and he turned over in his bed.

'Good night, Mr Smith, sleep well.'

'What was that all about?' enquired the staff nurse from the desk.

'The patient has now been reunited with his dentures.'

'Thank Heaven for that. We can all get some peace now.' I tip-toed out of the ward.

* * *

The patient sat upright on his trolley. Both his arms were strapped round his chest, his shirt was covered in vomit, and his trousers were soaked in urine. He was drunk. There are several types of drunks: happy drunks, sad drunks, silent drunks and violent drunks, and if this patient's injuries had not been so severe he would have been classified as the violent type. He was in an aggressive mood, and in spite of a barrage of four-letter words directed at the doctor and nurses, they still carried on in the best traditions of their profession. Sister Sue, who was on duty, was trying to discover how he had injured himself.

'How did you manage to injure your arms?' she asked.

'Mind your own bleeding business,' came the reply.

'Look, we're trying to help you.'

'Piss off.'

The doctor turned red. His patience was wearing thin. He looked at Sue, gave a shrug and started to fill in an X-ray form. Sue gave him a wink and turned once again to the patient.

In the quiet silky voice she could adopt when necessary, she started to plead with him.

'Now, Sir, you must tell us about your injuries. After all, we are here to serve you, and we cannot work to the maximum of our efficiency unless we have your full co-operation. We have our own reputation to uphold, and the public expect a high standard of patient care in this hospital.'

The patient looked bemused, the doctor's face gave a twitch, and I suppressed a smile.

'Won't you please help us?' Sue gave him one of her special smiles that I had seen before, the sort that would charm Satan himself. 'Please ...' she went on.

'Well I've been on the piss ...'

'I would never have guessed,' said Sue.

'... I tripped over a kerbstone and fell forward on my arms.'

The doctor passed me a pink X-ray form, shook his head and retreated to the staff room. Sue turned to the patient again. 'Now Sir,' she said, and pointed at me. 'This gentleman upholds the high traditions of this hospital, and he's going to take you for an X-ray. And if by any chance my staff have any more abuse from you, I'll stuff your f...ing mouth full of cotton wool. Take him away Walter.'

There was a look of amazement on the patient's face as I wheeled him along the corridor to the X-ray Department, where he joined the queue. But I was expecting too much to think that the patient's attitude had changed. I stayed with him while he was being X-rayed, and his profanities continued as the radiographer tried to position his arms. It was a relief to finally return him to the Casualty Department where he could await the results of his X-rays. They were not long in coming. Sister Sue came out of the doctor's room holding the plates up to view them from the overhead lighting.

'Deposit him in the Fracture Clinic, Walter.'

'Yes, Sister.'

Sue was about to walk away when there was another burst of abuse from the patient.

'Look, I pay my National Health for you buggers to look after me. What's happened to my arms?'

'You've fractured both of them.'

'Well, what does that mean?'

'It means, Sir, that you are going to have great difficulty wiping your arse every time you go for a shit over the next six weeks.'

She hurried away without waiting for an answer.

* * *

I knocked at the door of the small side room and pushed my way in with a tray of tea that Sister Sue had requested. Apart from Sue there was the doctor, along with a woman and a man who was obviously her husband. The woman was sobbing as she rocked too and fro clutching a baby in her arms. She held it close to her breast, and the tears streaming down her face were falling on the child. The tears were for the baby. It was dead.

The trauma of finding her daughter, who was only a few weeks old, dead in her cot had overwhelmed her. She could not grasp the fact that the child had died.

'She must still be alive, it couldn't possibly have happened to her.'

Her voice broke through the sobs that echoed round the room. She had been holding the baby for over two hours now, and in spite of the comforting words from her husband, the doctor and Sister Sue, she would not part with the child.

Sadly, cot deaths were not unknown in the Casualty

Department. It was another aspect of the work that the staff had to deal with, but it always left a deep well of sorrow in the hearts of the people involved.

It was much later, when the parents had returned home, that I picked up the child from the trolley and cradled her in my arms. She was still wrapped in her shawl and I was taking her to the mortuary. It was a late Summer evening, and visiting time was just finishing. Small groups of people stood outside the main doors engaged in conversation as I passed. The sight of me in a white coat holding a small baby seemed to catch their eye, and there were smiles as I made my way past them.

'Is that doctor going to make that baby better?' a small girl asked her mother.

Dear God. I wish I could have.

Chapter 6

More Accidents and Emergencies

"My soul sit thou a patient looker-on; Judge not the play before the play is done: Her plot has many changes every day Speaks a new scene; the last act crowns the play."

As the years passed the workload of the Casualty Department increased dramatically. The staff did their best to cope in what was an outdated building, and it was a relief to learn that plans for a new wing had been approved. The time between approval and actual building however, would be years rather than months if the money was not available. But everyone carried on optimistically, always with hope in their hearts that their conditions would improve.

As fast as one problem was solved in the department another arose. Even the political upheaval in East Africa had its affects. Over a very short period there was a great influx of Asians in the city. Very few could speak English, and at times it was difficult to assess what was wrong with them. It was their custom at that early period to arrive in groups to support the sick patient, and the person in the group who could speak the best English would act as the spokesman or woman. It was not unknown for the whole group to request a medical check-up, as they had prior information that the National Health Service was free in their new country, so why not use it? Most requests for treatment, however, were brief and to the point, like: 'My wife can't shit' or 'My piss hurts'. Perhaps their terminology had been acquired locally.

'Can I help you?' I asked one group late on a Saturday

night through the glass screen on the counter. There was a group of six men, and it was just after midnight. I wondered what could be wrong.

There was a worried exchange of words between them, and some gesturing in an excited manner, as I stood patiently waiting. I was relieving Ron, the night receptionist, who had gone to the dining room for his break, and I was on the desk by myself. After a time the group seemed to come to a decision, and they pushed forward a small Indian whose head appeared just over the top of the counter. I bent down to talk to him.

'Can I help you?' I repeated.

He put his lips to the aperture in the glass screen and spoke. His stream of words were completely unintelligible to my ear.

'Me ... end ... dee ... dee ... dee ...' Or at least that's what it sounded like.

I paused and thought deeply about the situation. As we had no interpreter amongst the staff, I knew there was no one that I could appeal to. I assumed that someone in the group needed some help, whoever he might be. I repeated my question again through the glass screen, slowly this time.

'Can ... I ... help ... you?'

The same words came through the aperture on curry-laden breath.

'Me ... end ... dee ... dee ... dee ...'

Then I had an inspired thought. How stupid of me, I had the obvious answer. Slowly, I said again: 'You ... want ... a... cup ... of ... tea?' And pointing to the tea machine in the corner of the waiting room, I went on: 'You ... get ... it ... over ... there.'

The response was not encouraging. There was a babble of voices and a committee meeting which produced another spokesman, who was much taller. I didn't have to bend over the desk to talk to him. He spoke in a slightly lower tone changing the dee's into tee's: 'Me ... end ... tee ... tee ... tee ...'

I was about to give up when Ron arrived back from his break.

'Help me, Ron. I can't make out what these people want. I don't understand a word they're saying.'

'Don't worry, Walter, it's the glass screen. Go outside and talk to them, you'll understand them better.'

I walked outside to the waiting room and stood surrounded by the Indians. The second spokesman, gesturing with both hands, burst out in a rapid voice once again.

'Me ... end ... tee ... tee ... tee ...'

I took a deep breath and tried again, this time in a very loud voice, waving my hands as I spoke.

'YOU ... SPEAK ... VERY ... SLOWLY ... AND ... TELL ... ME ... WHAT ... IS ... WRONG.'

The answer came back in the same vein.

'MY ... FRIEND ... HE ... HAS ... VD ...'

I went back behind the counter, and Ron looked up from his newspaper.

'Did you find out what was wrong?' he asked.

'Yes. His friend has V.D.'

'I'm not surprised,' he said, turning to the racing page. 'It's all that curry they eat.'

It took quite a while for some of the ethnic groups to realise that the Accident and Emergency Department was not an all-embracing medical service for general use; that the magic three nines dialled on the phone for an ambulance would not give them a free ride to their own GP's surgery; and that ambulances should not be used to bring in patients suffering from toothache. The Ambulance Service was hard-pressed at the best of times, and fortunately this abuse did taper off with time.

Some Indian patients had their own type of remedies to treat their casualties. Burns and scalds were sprinkled with curry powder, and this caused great problems to the patient concerned when the staff had to treat the infected area. They brought with them strange pills and potions that were impossible to identify, which they had purchased from some back-street doctor at exorbitant prices. The initial difficulties in dealing with the ethnic minorities were slowly overcome as the language barriers were broken down, with the introduction of new staff, who with patience and understanding helped them with their special needs.

* * *

There must be a very thin line in our statute book between stealing a car and taking it away without the owner's permission. There were many occasions when young joyriders ended up in the Casualty Department. Sadly some were B.I.D's (brought in dead) as were the innocent victims of their crimes, who had also lost their lives in the incident. The damage done to motor vehicles could perhaps be repaired, but human lives could not be renewed.

Joe Boggins was such a character. Aged seventeen, he had been in trouble many times, and he was well known by the local police. Joe decided one night to take his friend joy-riding. He stole a car outside a house and drove off at high speed along the main road on the outskirts of the city. While taking a bend too fast, Joe lost control and hit a telegraph pole. Tragically, his friend Bill was killed while Joe escaped with minor injuries, and he was brought into the Casualty Department by ambulance. It was just after I had taken him to the X-ray Department that a well-dressed man stopped me in the corridor and asked me where he was, as he wanted to see him. As there was a death involved in the incident, and I knew that the police, who were on their way, wanted to interview Joe, I was reluctant to give him any information. So I fetched Sister.

'Are you a relative?' she asked.

'Yes, I'm the father.'

'He's gone for an X-ray. Walter will take you to him.'

I led him along the corridor where Joe Boggins lay on a trolley waiting in the queue. Joe was having a conversation with a pretty girl in a wheelchair nearby, who had injured her leg, and he was evidently enjoying himself, for we could hear him laughing as we approached. It was hard to realise that he had been involved in a fatal accident just over an hour before. He didn't see us coming, and I addressed him from the back of the trolley.

'Your father's here, Joe.'

Joe stopped laughing and he turned round. The colour drained from his face, and he seemed to freeze and stiffen as he lay on his back. I wondered what had caused him to change so suddenly, when the man with me pushed me aside and nearly knocked me over. Reaching Joe, he grabbed him round the neck and started shaking him, trying to drag him off the trolley. I thought at the time that it was a rather strange way for a father to greet his son who had been injured in an accident.

'You murdering bastard!' the man cried. 'I told our Bill never to go out with you, but he wouldn't listen. Now you've killed him so I'm going to kill you.'

Oh, not in here, I thought. Joe was now going blue in the face as the man's hands pressed deeper round Joe's throat. I started yelling along the corridor for help, and the radiographer must have pressed the panic button because the alarm bell started ringing. The only action I could think of was to jump on the man's back and put my arms tightly round his neck. It seemed to have some effect; as I pulled his head back he took his hands off Joe, and tried to pull mine away.

'Leave me alone!' he shouted. 'I'll finish this murdering sod. My son would be alive now if it wasn't for him.'

I had a brief glimpse of the girl in the wheelchair getting up and dashing along the corridor, forgetting about her injured leg, and the other patients waiting for X-rays who could walk following her. The man was now struggling and trying to shake me off his back, but I still managed to cling to him. Help in the shape of two doctors and some porters arrived on the scene.

'What's going on?' someone shouted.

'For God's sake, help me, he's trying to murder this patient.'

The whole affair was now like a rugby scrum, with four men trying to heave the man away from Joe. Then someone tackled the man round his legs and he collapsed backwards on to the floor with me underneath him. I let the doctors and porters complete the operation and hold the man until the police arrived on the scene and took him away, still struggling and making threats against Joe, who was returned to Casualty so the red marks on his neck could be checked.

An hour later I made a statement to the police, who were now investigating the affair. Over a cup of tea I pointed out that the man had misled Sister by saying that he was the father, but forgetting to mention that he was Bill's father, not Joe's.

'Are you hurt, Walter?' Sister asked.

'Only my pride,' I answered. 'May I have another cup of tea please?'

* * *

The attitude of the doctors in Casualty towards the nursing staff and the porters varied. Some were very friendly, others would acknowledge you with a nod in passing, and some would completely ignore you. Many were local GPs who worked part-time, but they were always supported by the housemen and consultants.

One of the orthopaedic surgeons was an oriental gentleman by the name of Mr Wong. He was a man who was highly respected for his skills, but he did not suffer fools gladly, and it showed in his consulting room when he was dealing with some of his patients. His mode of dress after work was, to say the least unusual, as he wore denim trousers and tank-tops, and he looked like a member of one of the Chinese Tongs.

He was very interested in purchasing a new BMW, and after a test drive he turned to the salesman, who was not at all impressed by the appearance of this minute figure, and told him that he would buy it.

The salesman, still rather suspicious of this roughly dressed person, looked down at this small prospective buyer and, in a sarcastic voice, said:

'And how do you intend to pay for it, Sir?'

'Why, cash of course,' came the answer.

Not giving up easily, the salesman went on: 'I suppose you're in the take-away business?'

'Yes,' said Mr Wong. 'I take away arms, legs and anything else that causes trouble.'

* * *

Some of the visitors to Casualty were real nuisances. They wasted the time of the staff, and their complaints were not of a genuine nature. But even so, they were subjected to the usual routine checks by a doctor. Amongst our prime examples was a patient called Victor, a young man in his early twenties who seemed to spend most of his time reporting sick with all sorts of strange complaints. His visits were always made late at night, and he used the excuse that he was unable to get his own GP to visit him, which was hardly surprising.

After being checked one night by a doctor for some obscure illness, and told that he was in fairly good condition, he was discharged and told to go home. It was then that Victor began his usual tirade against the world in general, and the uncaring staff in our Casualty Department in particular.

'I'm not wanted in this world,' he went on. 'I'm going to end it all when I leave here.'

'Don't be silly,' Sister advised. 'Go home and have a good night's sleep. You'll feel better in the morning.' She had heard threats like that before.

But Victor did not go home that night. The new wing of the hospital was nearing completion at that time, and Victor, after clambering through the dark interior, somehow managed to gain access to the roof, which was several storeys high. As the building was in a deserted part of the hospital, he must have been there quite a long time before he made his presence known. The Casualty Department was alerted when a man approached the reception desk and waited his turn in the queue. 'Can I help you?' Ron the receptionist asked.

'I'm sorry to trouble you,' the man replied nonchalantly, 'but there's a chap on top of one of your buildings who says he's going to jump off. I thought I'd let you know.' And without waiting for an answer, he about turned and walked away.

The panic button was pressed, and on instructions from the senior nursing officer, the Police were alerted, then the Ambulance Service, followed by the Fire Service. In the search that followed, it took about ten minutes to locate Victor, and another ten minutes to identify him. But to set up the talk-down procedures it took much longer. If anyone climbed up and approached Victor, he would lean further over the scaffolding and tell them to go back. Like an actor, he held centre stage and seemed to be enjoying it. He ignored all the pleas and persuasion to come down from his lofty perch as he stood defiant, a black figure against the night sky.

Fred the ambulance man was getting tired of the waiting game, as he should have been off-duty nearly two hours ago.

'I wish he would make up his mind and jump, then we could all go home. They should send for his mother, she would frighten the Hell out of him. She certainly scared me the last time I took him home in my ambulance.'

Perhaps it was Fred's idea that sparked off what happened next. Twenty minutes later a police car arrived and out stepped a middle-aged woman. She was wearing a headscarf that almost hid the rollers in her hair, but failed to cover some at the side of her face, which dangled like lone earrings. She still wore a pair of slipper, and judging from her mode of dress, she had been aroused from her sleep in a hurry. The Police Inspector in charge of the operation went and spoke to her, and gesturing upwards they lifted their eyes in the general direction of Victor. The woman brushed off the offer of a loud hailer and walked to the base of the building. Hands on hips, she looked upwards again.

'What the bloody hell do you think you are doing up there?' she yelled. 'Getting me out of bed in the early hours of the morning! Get down here right away.'

There was no reply from Victor, and for once he stopped talking. She who must be obeyed had spoken. His mother took another deep breath and filled her lungs.

'If I come up there I'll break your bloody neck, causing me all this trouble. Besides, you know you've got to go to work tomorrow.'

There was silence from above and the figure of Victor drew back from the edge of the scaffolding.

'Are you coming down then?'

'Alright, mam,' came the meek answer. 'Only because I love you.'

‘I’ll kill the bugger when I get him back home,’ his mother went on to the Police Inspector. ‘I had enough trouble with his old man when he was alive.’

The sheepish figure of Victor finally emerged from the building. The fire engine with the high turn-table ladder drove off, the ambulance crew started to report back by radio to their control centre, while Victor and his mother were driven away in a police car. Peace reigned once more.

‘Goodnight, Fred,’ I called to the ambulance driver. ‘Victor will be in trouble when he gets home.’

‘It will be nothing like what I’ve got coming to me from my old woman. I’m over three hours late already. It’s the spare room for me tonight.’

* * *

The Accident and Emergency Department was always changing its procedures as necessity dictated, to try and keep up with the growing pressures. The Flying Squad, which consisted of a team of doctors and nurses who were on stand-by and were used for outside emergencies, was reorganised. A staff nurse was detailed from every shift for what was known as triage duty; this was to assess the condition of incoming patients who had come in for treatment.

One factor that did not change was the violence. It started on the city streets and spilled over into the hospital. Members of opposing factions carried on their fights in the waiting room when they brought their injured in for treatment. They had no respect for the staff or for the other innocent patients waiting for treatment. The police always gave priority for the hospital’s call for help, but a great degree of damage usually took place before they arrived on the scene.

Rather than leave a sick or elderly patient alone while

they were waiting for treatment, or for an ambulance to take them back home, I was often requested to stay with them in the cubicle area, where the only privacy offered to a patient were the curtains drawn round their trolley. The conversations from the other cubicles could be heard loud and clear.

I sat listening to one of the new doctors trying to make sense of old Steve, one of the regulars who was stone deaf, and he was making hard work of it. He finished up shouting for all to hear.

'Are you regular?' the doctor yelled.

'Eh?'

'Are you regular in your habits?'

'Oh aye.'

'How many times do you go>'

'Twice a week.'

'Twice a week? That's not very often.'

'I can't afford to go any more.'

'What do you mean?'

'The beer's too expensive these days.'

'I'm talking about your bowels.'

'I gave up playing bowls years ago,'

The more intimate details of a girl's sex life no longer remained a secret to the patients in the surrounding cubicles as the doctor questioned her.

'When did you have your last period?' he asked.

'I'm not sure. It must have been two months ago.'

'Are you married?'

'No.'

'I have to ask. Have you had any sexual relations lately?'

'What do you mean?'

'Well have you been out with a boyfriend?'

'I don't have one.'

'You must have been with a man. I think you're pregnant.'

There was a brief pause.

'Well, I did go out for a ride in a car with a chap from the office.'

'When was that?'

'About three months ago.'

'Did anything happen?'

'Yes.'

'What?'

'We ran into a ditch.'

* * *

With the advent of the holiday period, and the desire for that all-important tan to show our friends, some people, mostly members of the younger generation, thought it necessary to revert to using sun-beds – with disastrous results. One weekend two young girls, with their skins the colour of lobsters and in great pain, made their own way to the hospital. The clothes they were wearing were causing them great distress simply by being in contact with their skin. They had exposed most of their bodies to the ultra violet rays from the lamps. The tears streaming down their faces indicated their distress, and they were also afraid of what their parents reactions would be. They had to be informed, as the girls were both admitted to the Burns Unit of the hospital.

In spite of all the warnings about the dangers of sunburn, the Casualty Department still had many patients seeking advice after they had returned from their Summer holidays. Some of them suffered from blistered skin, and a few of the female patients, who had been topless, must have been in agony. With the possibility of infection from such burns, the staff always referred such cases to the specialist concerned.

* * *

As the years passed the number of drug addicts in the city increased, and although there was a centre where they could get help, when they were in trouble they were invariably brought into Casualty. Some patients were found lying in the street, or behaving strangely. They were not the easiest people to deal with. Many were violent as the effects wore off, and others were in a euphoric state of mind, in a world of their own. Some were victims of their own weaknesses and died from an overdose. Sadly, they never seemed to realise how much misery they had bequeathed to their relatives and friends.

The guests drinking at the bar of one of the city's largest hotels were surprised one Saturday night by a very pretty girl who made a sweeping entrance. The surprise arose from the fact that all she was wearing was a diaphanous nightdress. The loud conversation fell to a hush as she walked in, and even the hotel staff, who had witnessed many strange events during their work, were shocked. As ever, in true British spirit, the hotel manager, not being sure if his guest was drunk or suffering from some mental blackout, put a coat round her and escorted her back to her room. There he found a syringe on the bedroom floor and a piece of screwed up paper with a few grains of a white substance inside. It was then he suspected she had been taking drugs and, not knowing exactly what to do to safeguard the reputation of the hotel, he phoned the police, who advised him to call and ambulance and take her to hospital. So she ultimately arrived at Casualty, and the ambulance men revealed her story.

The girl's behaviour was most erratic, and apart from discovering that her name was Alma, no further information was forthcoming. So after examination by a doctor, she was put on a trolley and placed in a side room. Her translucent nightdress was changed for a paper gown, that was considered to be less revealing. After a time Alma became more relaxed and appeared to be asleep, and the nurse who had been constantly watching her was withdrawn, as the department began to fill up with more urgent cases.

It was some time afterwards when things started to happen. A local resident phoned to say that a naked woman was standing under a lamp-post opposite his house, in a street adjoining the hospital. Was it anything to do with those drunken medical students who were always causing trouble, he wanted to know? The telephone operators at the hospital receive some very strange messages and this one worked its way through the channels. It was left for the porters to investigate. Starting in the Casualty Department, it was soon discovered that one of Sister's patients was missing. Yes, it was Alma!

How she had made her escape was a mystery, as the staff had been systematically checking on her as they worked. They were concerned about the patient's condition, so the police were informed. In the meantime, the porters formed a posse to go and look for her. The sheriff in charge was the shift leader, Danny, and he issued orders, allocating various territories for us to search.

He turned to me. 'You scour the local pubs, Walter, and make enquiries.' He went on: 'I don't want my lads to go inside or I shan't see the drunken buggers again tonight. We'll split up and search the rest of the area.' With that he mustered his posse and set off, trailed by his own contingent consisting of Big Albert, Little Don and a porter known to everyone for some obscure reason as the Brain.

As the errand boy for the department, I knew the local pubs well through fetching cigarettes, crisps, biscuits and mineral water for the staff when the hospital dining room was closed. I was sure that Alma would not be found inside any of them, or someone would have reported her whereabouts by now, but I went inside and looked round, refusing offers from regulars to stay and have a drink. There was no sign of Alma.

Seeing a man walking his dog, I stopped and asked him if he had seen a naked lady about. He gave me a strange look and enquired if his wife had left her bathroom curtains open again. The search so far had proved futile, and I had just decided to return to Casualty when Danny's voice yelled from the darkness, 'Catch her, Walter ... catch her!'

Coming to me out of the gloom was Alma, bare-footed and completely naked. She was running at a tremendous pace. It was doubtful whether under ordinary circumstances I would have caught her, but she held her head high as she ran and probably did not see me. A rugby tackle was out of the question, so I met her head on, our two bodies making an impact. It could be described as an astronomical collision, like two heavenly bodies meeting, as I saw stars from the blow, and I came off worse. But I managed to get my arms round her waist in spite of her struggles and cling on to her. Danny, puffing and panting, came up from the rear, followed by his merry men.

'Thank God you caught her, we've been chasing her round the bloody block, and I'm knackered,' he said.

'If you don't give me a hand to hold her, you're going to lose her again,' I replied, as Alma was still struggling to get away.

'We'd better cover her up,' Danny went on, and turning to Big Albert, the tallest of the porters, he said 'Put your overall over her vital parts before we take her back.'

Reluctantly, Big Albert agreed, but it was no easy operation, as Alma was not in a very co-operative mood. Kicking and struggling, she was as slippery as an eel, and she was making giggling noises as we tried to hold her.

'Grab her arms and legs,' said Danny, 'we'll carry her.'

The porters duly obliged and they managed to lift Alma

into a horizontal position with Big Albert's white coat covering her. It was then that the Great British Public came on the scene. There was just one couple to begin with, and then there was a crowd that seemed to appear from nowhere. We moved slowly through them, and I could hear the questions.

'Has she been raped ...?'

'Is she dead ...?'

Danny took a deep breath. 'The silly sods,' he said. 'Let's get her out of here. We can take a short cut through the Maternity Wing, and we can borrow a blanket and trolley from there.'

With the struggling Alma, we slowly made our way along the road, still followed by a group of onlookers, and with Big Albert still trying to cover Alma with his overall. Little Don, who was holding her legs at the front of the procession, stopped suddenly.

'What's the matter?' asked Danny.

'Is it raining?' Don enquired.

'Don't be daft, of course not.'

'Then she must be pissing over me,' said little Don.

The Maternity Wing of the hospital stood apart from the main building on the opposite side of the road, and was joined to it by an underground corridor. Stella, the receptionist on duty, looked up from behind her desk in surprise as we burst in through the doors. We made for the trolley that was used for incoming emergencies, placed the almost naked girl on it and covered her with a blanket.

'What's happening?' asked Stella. 'Is she expecting a baby.'

'No, but she will be if we let her run about in this state,' said Danny. 'Hold her down while we get her back to Casualty'.

Our return was greeted with sighs of relief from Sister and the staff, and the police were informed that she had been found. All was well again. Little Don, however, was not at all happy.

'Do I get a new pair of trousers? She's pissed all over this pair.'

Danny was not impressed. 'Consider yourself lucky,' he said. 'You might have been covered in shit.'

* * *

When the doors of the Casualty Department opened, the staff were never surprised by the unexpected. Tonight they revealed a young man about five feet tall sandwiched in between two six-foot policemen who towered over him.

'Would you book him in while I go and have a word with Sister?' said one of the officers.

'What's wrong with him?' I enquired.

'He's been bitten by a dog.'

'Where?' I asked.

'Can't you tell by the position of his hands?'

A closer look revealed a pair of blood-stained trousers torn at the front, and the young man's hands positioned between his legs.

'Was he bitten on the testicles?'

'I don't think so, but it must have been very close. That's why we brought him straight here.'

'You shouldn't have sent that bloody dog after me,' said the young man.

'You shouldn't have been breaking into that shop, and trying to get away.'

'I'm going to sue the police for this,' said the victim.

'It's no good you suing us. Sue the dog,' said the officer.

Over the years a great many people suffering from dog bites came to us for treatment. Some had serious lacerations, and these patients had to be admitted for further treatment. These incidents caused great distress when they happened to children, and it must have had a profound effect on their future attitudes towards animals.

I don't know if some dogs go mad at times, but in the majority of cases, the pets that had turned on their owners and other people, had been in the family for years. There was a sense of disbelief from some owners that such an incident could happen. Patients were usually given an anti-tetanus injection as part of the treatment, although this was perhaps a precaution against future dog bites, rather than the existing one.

* * *

Wife battering was almost regarded as a sport by some husbands, and their victims were frequent visitors to Casualty. Violence of this nature can never be justified, whatever the reasons put forward by the perpetrators. Some of these patients had extensive injuries, but refused to take any action against the men responsible. One of the common causes was drink, but sometimes the assault could be due to a trivial domestic episode that was blown out of all proportion.

Very often the husband would attend the hospital after his wife had been admitted. No doubt suffering from a guilty conscience, and overcome by remorse, he would demand to see her. The wife's reaction was usually one of fear, and she would implore the staff not to let him into the ward. When the husband was refused entry this could be the cue for a violent confrontation, often leading to police action.

It has also been known for incidents of this nature to happen to a very different kind of victim.

Charlie Moggins made his way to the reception desk one evening.

'Can I see a doctor, please?' he enquired.

He was an upright man about six-feet tall with very broad shoulders. He looked the type who could be found playing in the front of a rugby scrum or weight-lifting in a gymnasium.

'What's wrong, Sir?' Alf the receptionist asked.

'I think I may have broken my ribs. I fell over.'

'You look as though you've been run over,' said Alf.

Charlie did look in a poor way. His right eye was swollen and turning red, his face was bruised and cut, and he was holding his hand over his rib cage as though he was having difficulty in breathing. After he was booked in I took him to the treatment cubicles and handed him over to the staff nurse.

'Can you help this patient to get undressed, Walter. He looks as though he may need some help,' she said.

He certainly did need some help. After I removed his shirt the bruises on his body were revealed. They covered the upper part of his torso and the red patches extended round his back.

'It must have been some fall you had,' I remarked.

Some patients relate strange stories to cover up how they came by their injuries, and never reveal the true facts. Charlie evidently belonged to that group. His private life was his own affair, but it always helped the staff when patients were honest with them; after all, they were not there to sit in moral judgement on the people who came in for treatment. As I assisted him to climb on to the trolley and covered him with a blanket, he groaned with pain. The staff nurse then took over, and I returned to the reception desk to find Alf waiting for me.

'Can you take this lady through to Mr Moggins?' he asked. 'It's his wife.' And he pointed to a small woman who stood on the other side of the counter, and whose head just came up to the aperture in the glass screen.

'The nurse is with him at the moment doing his observations, but I'll go and tell him you are here.'

There were times when I found it difficult to communicate with some patients, as my words never seemed to get through, but this was not the case with Charlie Moggins. The six little words I uttered had a profound effect on him.

'Your wife is here, Mr Moggins.'

His reaction was that of a desperate man. He shot upright on the trolley, almost knocking to the floor the sphygmomanometer that the nurse was using to take his blood pressure. His face went a paler shade of yellow beneath his bruises, and he made an effort to climb off the trolley, but was restrained by the nurse.

'What's the matter with you?' she asked.

'Don't let her get near me, she'll finish me off,' came the reply.

'But she must be anxious about your injuries from the fall.'

'Fall, be buggered, it was that old cow hitting me with her walking stick that she keeps in the corner of the room. You've got to protect me.'

'Protect you?'

'I'm one of those battered husbands that you read about.'

'Bloody hell!' said the staff nurse. 'I've heard everything now. I'll go and have a word with Sister. Stay with the patient, Walter, I'll go and fetch her.'

Sister, as all good sisters do, started to reassure the patient. 'You don't have to see your wife if you don't want to,' she explained. 'Do you want to report this incident to the police?'

'No. Just keep her away from me while I make my escape. I'm pissing off.'

'You must stay here and let the doctor check you over. He'll probably want to send you for an X-ray.'

But Charlie had other ideas. He already had one leg in

his trousers and was struggling to get the other one in.

'If you are going to take your own discharge, you will have to sign a form to the effect that you are refusing treatment,' said Sister.

'I don't mind. If she gets her hands on me again I shall be signing my own death warrant. Just give me a head start.'

Sister shrugged. 'Alright, Staff Nurse, if he wants to go, we can't stop him.' She turned to Charlie Moggins. 'I think you are being very silly.'

'You don't know my wife,' said Charlie.

When Alf broke the news to Mrs Moggins, all five foot three of her, that her beloved had eluded her, she was not very pleased, and she became more incensed when she was told that she could not search the department to look for him. She started complaining that she was the victim of some conspiracy by the National Health Service. But by this time Charlie had melted into the sunset, while his wife, after a great argument, was escorted off the premises by two porters, who were taking no chances with her when they learned that she was violent.

I never did find out what happened to Charlie.

* * *

I watched Claudia the radiographer as she pushed her portable X-ray machine along the corridor. It was an awkward piece of equipment and she was struggling to control the monster, as it seemed to have a mind of its own. She stopped for a moment, exhausted by her efforts, and I went over to her.

'Do you want a hand, Claudia?' I asked.

'Thanks, Walter, this thing drains you of all your energy.' 'Where are we going?'

'I don't quite know, I'm looking for a patient who was injured when a building fell on him.'

'Have you tried the mortuary?'

'He must be somewhere around. I've got his X-ray form.'

'What's his name?'

'It looks like Smith, but the doctor's writing is atrocious.'

'There have been two Smiths booked in but they've gone home now. Can I borrow your X-ray form? I'll try and find him for you.'

'Thanks, Walter.'

Ron, the night receptionist who had just come on duty, gave me a blank look when I asked him if he knew the whereabouts of a patient named Smith who was suffering from injuries through a building collapsing on him.

'I've just come on duty,' he replied. 'I don't have any details of a patient by that name.'

Further enquiries of the nursing staff about the missing patient yielded no clues to his whereabouts. I began to wonder if Mr Smith really existed. Finally I made my way to Sister's office, knocked on the door and walked in. She looked up from the duty rota she was preparing. 'What is it, Walter?' she asked.

'I'm looking for a patient who was trapped in a building when it collapsed, Sister, and no one knows where he is. I want to take him for an X-ray.'

'No one's told me about the incident since I came on duty. Have you got his X-ray form?'

I passed it to her, and she looked closely at it.

'This is Dr Pill's writing. Let's see if he's in the office, perhaps he can explain. I want to know what's going on in the department.'

She swept out of the room and I followed at her heels as she made her way to the staff room. Dr Pill was there, sitting with his feet up on a small table and drinking a cup of coffee. Sister wasted no time in her approach.

'Why wasn't I informed about this patient?' she asked, and there was a hardness in her voice.

'What patient?' Dr Pill asked.

'The patient who was injured when a building fell on him.'

'A building fell on him? What are you talking about? I know nothing about such an incident.'

'It's your writing on the X-ray form, look at it. It says Mr Smith. Cause of injuries: house fell on him.' She handed him the form.

Dr Pill looked at it and slowly shook his head in disgust.

'That word is not house, it's horse. His horse fell on top of him when he was out riding this afternoon. The poor chap has been in the Fracture Clinic for about five hours waiting to have his leg put in plaster, and I wanted a re-X-ray done before I sent him home. He was here before you came on duty. You must teach your staff how to read, Sister.'

'And I would like to teach you doctors how to write.'

'If he had brought his horse in with him, I wouldn't have had all this trouble finding him,' I said.

* * *

'Can you give us a hand, Walter?' asked Mike, the ambulance-man who, along with his mate, was struggling to transfer a male patient on to a trolley. 'Be careful how you lift. I think it could be a fractured femur.'

By using the canvas sheet that the man was lying on, we managed to move him without causing him any further distress, and he was wheeled to the treatment area.

'You meet some bloody queer people in this world,' said Mike as he stood folding his blankets.

'What do you mean?' I asked.

'We had a 999 call to say that a man had fallen down the stairs from a house in the Stoney Lane district, and you know how posh those residences are. We got to the place in about five minutes. It was a great big house with a front door flanked with big pillars and potted plants, and we stood ringing the door bell for a long time. Nobody answered, so after a while we decided to go round the back of the house. We hammered on what must have been the kitchen door, and after some time a woman came. She confirmed that her husband had fallen down the stairs and injured himself. We followed her through the house and discovered him lying in the hall behind the front door. I turned to her and told her that we had wasted several minutes trying to get in, and had she heard us ringing the door bell. "Oh yes," she replied, "but I do expect you to use the tradesmen's entrance".'

* * *

'Thy never tell us,' said Ken. 'They must think that the portering staff are expendable, the way they treat us.'

We had just arrived at the ward with a male patient on a trolley, to find two nurses dressed in barrier clothing waiting for us outside the small side room. That usually meant that the patient we had handled was suffering from some infectious disease. We had been asked to accompany a nurse from Casualty and give her any necessary help, as she was a small girl, and Ken and I were there to do the lifting. She too was ignorant of the patient's symptoms. Ken turned to the staff nurse in charge and whispered, 'No one told us that we needed barrier clothing. We're not dressed to lift the patient.'

'It's alright, Ken, the patient will be able to move over on his own.'

It was only when we returned to Casualty that Ken discovered our patient was suffering from some form of hepatitis, which did not please him. Throughout the year, patients passed through the Accident and Emergency Department suffering from all sorts of strange illnesses, and whereas the medial and nursing staff were familiar with these diseases and took the necessary precautions, no one seemed to bother to warn the portering staff about the dangers of cross-infection. With the advent of AIDS and all the national publicity surrounding it, procedures started to change. Blood samples carried by the porters to the Haematology Department were no longer carried loosely in their overall pockets, but were now put in plastic envelopes for safer transportation. Gloves were used for handling urine samples.

The letters AIDS didn't mean much to the portering staff in the early days, but as publicity and warnings increased, they inspired a degree of fear. George, the Father of the Lodge, knew all about AIDS.

'It's not new. They've been doing it for years,' said George.

'Doing what?' young David asked.

'This A.I.D. thing.'

David wouldn't give up. 'Well, what does it mean then?'

'Didn't your mother teach you anything?' George went on. 'It means Artificial Insemination by Donor. You know they get the what-do-you-call-it from the male organ, and inject it in the female's you-know-where, and Bingo ... well you know what I'm talking about, don't you?'

'Yes, cows.'

'Cows?'

'I saw it on television. They were doing it on a farm, and I bet the bull wasn't too happy about it.'

'You're bloody hopeless,' said George, and walked away in disgust.

The nursing staff in the early days were asked to keep secret the details of any patient diagnosed as an AIDS victim when they were sent to ward, so as not to cause any panic or concern to the rest of the patients. But as time progressed there was a greater understanding of patients' needs, and fear of the disease lessened. But there was no let-up in the precautions taken by the staff who had to deal with these unfortunate people. Fear of the unknown plays a large part in our lives, and this particularly applied to some people who at last plucked up courage to consult a doctor after suffering months of uncertainty. Fear of cancer could cause great distress, when there might have been a simple explanation for their symptoms; and those so-called pains in the chest that turned out to be a stomach upset often helped lift a black cloud of fear from people's lives.

The Accident and Emergency Department must have been a chaotic place at first sight to the incoming patient, with the waiting room at times strewn with human debris, drunks misbehaving, children crying, and unabated foul language. But it was there to serve the people of the city, open every day all through the year.

We complained about the place, we criticised it, we sometimes even hated it, but we couldn't do without it.

Chapter 7

Trauma

No man ever offended his own conscience, but, first or last it was avenged upon him for it.

It was a quiet night and a proliferation of porters sat out of sight on a bench at the end of the corridor. George, the Father of the Lodge, was relating tales about his wartime experiences when he was stationed with the army in India, and he had just reached the climax of an amorous adventure with a member of the opposite sex. Young David, the newest member of the group, sat listening open-mouthed. The Bishop sat quietly reading, with his head buried in a book, while the other members of the group sat stretched out and appeared to be dozing.

'...and so,' George went on, 'after one night with me, she threw caution to the winds and followed me everywhere.'

'What about her parents?' David asked.

'Oh, they wanted to sell her to me, but I didn't think she was worth ten rupees.'

'Why do some Indian women have red spots on their foreheads?' David asked.

'That means that they used to work in a brothel,' George said, giving me a wink.

'We get a lot of them in here,' said David.

'Well, don't ask them about it. They get a bit touchy on the subject. Now I remember when I was in Calcutta ...'

Sister's voice from the end of the corridor interrupted the rest of the story. 'Porter please ... Porter please ...'

I stood up and stretched myself. 'I'll go,' I said. I'd heard the Calcutta story several times before. The Bishop closed his book; he was clearly embarrassed by George's stories. 'I'll give you a hand,' he said.

Sister was waiting for us. 'Give the ambulance-men a hand, please.'

We had no need to ask where the help was needed, as a continuous high-pitched screaming sound came from the direction of the Ambulance Bay, and we hurried outside to find two ambulance-men struggling with a patient in the back of their vehicle. I could see the arms and legs of the man inside through the rear door. He was kicking and fighting off the efforts of the ambulance crew to lift him on to the nearby trolley, and as we climbed in the back, I noticed the blood-stained blanket that covered him.

'For God's sake, let's get him inside,' Mike the driver said. 'Get a leg each while we grab his arms, and watch out he doesn't kick you in the vulnerable areas. He almost ruined my wife's wedding present. Sister wants him in the Resuscitation Room.'

Lifting the now screaming, struggling man on to the trolley was no easy matter, and when we did succeed his struggles were just as violent.

'Can we use restraining straps?' one of the ambulance-men asked the doctor who had now joined us.

'Only as the last resort. I would rather manage without them at this stage.'

The patient was wheeled into the Resuscitation Room and the screams turned to moans. Undressing him proved to be difficult as he continued to struggle. The staff nurse started to remove his trousers that were now soaked in blood, while the Bishop and I stood at the head of the trolley, restraining him by holding his arms.

'Be careful,' warned Sister as the staff nurse finally removed the patient's trousers and dropped them on to the floor to reveal a bloody mess between the man's legs.

'What's happened to him?' I whispered to the ambulance-man who was standing beside me.

'He's cut his thingy off.'

'His thingy. What do you mean?'

'His joystick, his tool, or if you prefer it, his penis.'

'Oh my God!'

'For what it's worth, we've brought the missing bit with us. It's in the vomit bowl over there on ice.' He indicated with his hand. 'One thing's for sure, it's not going to be stitched back on. Take a look at it.'

'No thanks. What did he do it with?'

'We are not sure. He carried out the amputation in his garden shed, and it was likely done with a pair of garden shears. He apparently has a history of mental instability, and he has been in a mental institution recently. I gather he's some sort of religious maniac, according to his neighbours. He lives alone and no one seems to know much about his family.'

The patient was now being examined by a surgeon who had joined the casualty officer. He was not struggling so much now, which made our task easier. The Bishop was talking quietly to him in that soothing voice of his. Then, in between the moans from the trolley, there was a spate of words.

'What did he say?' I asked.

'He's quoting from the bible.'

The surgeon looked up from his examination in surprise. 'From the bible? What's he quoting then?'

'Matthew, chapter five, verses twenty-eight and twenty-nine.'

Everyone stopped and stared at the Bishop in surprise. They evidently knew nothing of his background, and most of the porters were regarded as ignorant clots by the medical staff on the grounds that they wouldn't be doing that sort of work otherwise.'

'Go on,' said the surgeon. 'Do you know them?'

There was a pause, and then, in between the patient's moans, the Bishop in a soft voice went on:

'But I say unto you that whosoever looketh on a woman to lust after her, hath committed adultery with her already in his heart.

'And if thy right eye offend thee pluck it out, and cast it from thee, for it is profitable for thee that one of thy members should perish, and not that the whole body should be cast into Hell.'

For one brief moment everyone stopped what they were doing, and several pairs of eyes now regarded the Bishop in a new light.

'That's bloody marvellous, laddie,' said the surgeon. 'You're in the wrong profession, you should be a bloody parson.' He sighed. 'I suppose it's another case of cherchez la femme. Right, let's get the patient up to the theatres. We'll do what we can but I don't think he'll ever be quite the same man again.'

The Bishop gave a sad little smile, and as we moved through the door I whispered in his ear, 'At least some one recognises your potential. We'll see you in Lambeth palace yet!'

* * *

The large car swung into the ambulance bay and stopped suddenly with a squeal of brakes. Danny the porter, who was sitting near me, looked up from the newspaper he was reading.

'Look at that silly sod pulling in there. Can't he read the notice "Ambulances Only"? It's big enough. Go and shift him, Walter.'

I made my way outside where the driver was struggling to get a man out of the nearside door.

'You can't park here, it's for ambulances only. Can't you see the signs?'

'I'm just bringing you a patient. I won't be long.'

The patient was acting somewhat strangely. He was coming out of the car backwards in a bent position, and seemed to have some difficulty walking. As the driver got back in his car and was preparing to move away, he gave a wave. 'See you later, Ronnie,' he shouted above the noise of the engine.

'Wait a minute, aren't you staying with him? He looks unsteady on his feet,' I said.

'No, I'll leave him in your caring hands.'

'What's happened to him?'

'He'll give you all the grim details.'

'I'd better get him a wheelchair.'

'Don't bother, he won't be in a hurry to sit down.' He put his foot down on the accelerator and shot away.

'Your friend's in a hurry,' I ventured.

'That bastard is no friend of mine, leaving me in the shit like this.' The man took a few unsteady steps towards the entrance.

'I'll get you a wheelchair to sit in, you can't walk very well.'

'I don't want one. Just point me in the direction of the Casualty Department and piss off.'

One learns quickly to soak up abuse from this type of patient. Argument usually makes confrontation worse, so I just pointed to the overhead sign which read "Accident and Emergency" and gave no answer. I watched him continue his strange walk as he staggered forward with his legs apart.

'He's walking like a pregnant duck,' Danny's voice echoed from behind me. 'What's wrong with him?'

'I don't know. He didn't say.'

'Ah well, go and have a cup of tea.'

It was some twenty minutes later when I came face to face with Ronnie again. Well, not quite face to face, as he was lying bottoms up on a trolley covered by a blanket.

'Take this patient down to X-ray and stay with him, Walter,' said the staff nurse as she pushed a pink X-ray form in to my hand. 'Bring him back again when he's ready.'

Joy, the night radiographer, was sitting reading a novel when I entered the department, and she looked up when I entered the door. 'What have you got for me?' she enquired.

'A male patient, but I don't know what's wrong with him.'

I handed her the form, and I saw the puzzled look on her face as she read it. 'This is a funny one,' she said.

'What's wrong?'

'He's got a foreign body in his anus. Ah well, it takes all sorts to make a world. Wheel him in, Walter, and stay while I do the X-ray. I don't want to be left on my own.'

About fifteen minutes later, I was standing with a silent Ronnie in the corridor outside the X-ray room, waiting for the plates, when Joy put her head round the door. 'Can you spare me a minute, Walter?' she asked.

I joined her inside the room. She was looking at one of the X-ray plates that was lit up in the viewing frame on the wall. 'What does this object look like that he's got stuck up his bum?' she asked, pointing to the plate.

I studied it for a few seconds. 'It looks like a small electric torch to me.'

She changed the plate for another one that was taken from another angle. As she did so, I could see the beginning of a smile on her lips as she viewed it. 'I think you may be right,' she said. 'Well, we'll soon find out. Take the patient back, Walter. It will come out in the wash.'

'Whatever it is, I think it will take more than washing to get it out.'

My return to Casualty must have been awaited with interest, as the X-ray plates were almost snatched out of my hand by Sister, who hurried with them to the staff room. I pushed the patient into a cubicle, and went looking for the staff nurse. I found her with the others, crowding round Ronnie's plates, that were being viewed on the wall.

'What's the object?' I enquired. 'Is it a small torch?'

They all looked at me, and I could see the smiles on their faces.

'Where have you been all your life?' one of the doctors asked. 'It's a vibrator.'

'A vibrator?'

'The type that some ladies use to ease themselves.'

'What's it doing up Ronnie's bottom?' I asked.

This was the cue for laughter, and my question remained unanswered. The doctor was gazing at the plates with great interest, and he turned to the rest of the staff.

'The batteries in the vibrator must be the long-life type. I'm almost certain that they are still working. We should write and congratulate the makers.'

'Probably Ever Ready, like the patient,' said a staff nurse. It was some time before I saw Danny the porter, and I stopped him as he passed me by.

'Danny, do you remember the man who you said walked like a pregnant duck?'

'Yes.'

'Well, he's going to lay an egg any moment now.'

Foreign bodies in bodily apertures were not confined to the male sex. The ladies had their share of problems too, and many strange objects had to be removed after they had become lodged in their sensitive areas. Various types of fruit and vegetables were extracted, and in one case a small cucumber. The patients involved in these incidents were usually highly embarrassed. Every precaution was taken to safeguard their privacy, but the clinical aspects of these situations were of great interest to the medical and nursing staff.

* * *

There was always a shortage of porters during certain periods of the year. In the Winter, when illness took its toll, and in the Summer, through holiday commitments. Although the porters were willing to work overtime, there were occasions when the hospital was desperately short staffed, and I was able to cover a whole range of duties. It was during one of these periods that the sight of an ambulance pulling into a bay made me instinctively move to a trolley and start pushing it towards the door. Andy the ambulance driver and his colleague Richard, who was always known as Big Dick to the staff, although he was only about five feet four, climbed out of the vehicle. Seeing me with the trolley, Andy waved me back with a sweep of his hand.

'We won't be needing that,' he said. 'Is Sister about?'

'She's in her office.'

'I'll have words with her,' he said and disappeared.

'What's the problem?' I asked Richard.

'We have two R.T.As in the back.'

'Why don't you bring them inside?'

'They're dead.'

'Oh.'

I pushed the trolley back to its previous position, and observed from afar as Sister and the doctor made their way to the rear of the ambulance. Richard opened the doors for them to look in the back, and I saw Sister turn her head and step back. There was some talk amongst the group, then Andy shut the doors, and then they all returned along the corridor towards me.

'Can you get me two porters, Walter?' Sister asked as she passed.

'I can get you one, Sister, he's the only person left in the lodge. It being holiday time, they are very short. Is there any way I can help?'

She paused. 'I don't think it's a very suitable job for you, Walter, there are two bodies to be taken to the mortuary.'

'I don't mind, I often go with the porters.'

She paused again. 'They're not a very nice sight. Get the other porter to help you and the ambulance-men to take them down, but remember, no one is forcing you to do this job. If you refuse when you see them, we shall think none of the worse of you.' She hurried away.

The only other porter available was the Bishop, who brought the keys of the mortuary with him. We made our way across the square to where the ambulance was waiting. He unlocked the mortuary doors and turned to the ambulance-men.

'Are we ready?' he asked.

'Where do you keep the barrier clothing?' Andy asked.

'Do we need it?'

'You certainly do.'

I looked at the Bishop, who did not answer, but led us all inside, where we donned gowns, gloves and caps.

'You'll need masks as well,' said Andy.

'Why all this bother?' I asked. 'I thought there were two R.T.As in the back?'

'That's right. You'll see why. Put your mask on.'

Suitably adorned, the Bishop and I followed him outside and he opened the rear doors of the ambulance. The smell from the interior permeated through out masks, choking us. It was acrid and acid-like, and caught the back of the throat with a great impact. It hung heavily in the air outside, and seemed to obscure the interior.

'God above!' I burst out, forgetting that the Bishop was with me. 'What the hell has happened to them?'

Two dark figures lay in the back of the ambulance, one on each side. Unrecognisable as human beings, they were charred and crisp. These shrivelled remains were unlike anything from this world. The heads had maintained their ovality, but they were like shrunken orbs without any signs of the eyes, ears, mouth or nose. The rest of their bodies were twisted with contorted limbs. One figure had part of an upright arm, twisted and blackened, raised in front of his head as if to protect his face. The remains were laid out on thick polythene sheeting, and were surrounded by pieces of burnt flesh that must have fallen off on the journey to the hospital.

'Did these come from an R.T.A.?' the Bishop asked.

'They did,' Andy replied. 'Their car burst into flames on impact and they had no chance. I only hope that the poor buggers died instantly and weren't burnt to death. We shall never know, shall we? This is the worst R.T.A. I've been involved in. Even the Police and the Fire Brigade were sickened at the sight when we recovered the bodies. Let's get them inside.'

Each of us holding a corner of the polythene sheeting, we lifted what remained of the two bodies into the mortuary and gently lowered them on to the floor, while the Bishop sorted out two empty chambers to put them in.

'Who are they?' I asked.

'We don't know. We're not even sure of their sex, but the Police think that at least one of the bodies is a man's by the type of wrist watch he was wearing. But it would be difficult to give a name to them individually, the state they're in, and it will be impossible for the relatives to identify them. I suppose it could be done through their dental charts.

The burnt bodies were placed on the trays from the interior chambers and as we lifted them, the black charred flesh flaked off with the movements of the polythene sheeting. It was not an easy task to get them inside the chamber. The partially raised arm of one of the corpses caught the top and a piece fell off, while the curled leg of the other was pushed back with rather dire results. But the task was finally completed and the Bishop recorded the arrival of two unidentified bodies in the register.

It was hard to realise that the remains we had handled were once human beings. It seemed that they had lost their identities as members of the human race, and the sadness that now overwhelmed me made me realise that only a short time ago they had been alive, perhaps laughing and joking as they travelled along. The Bishop stood alone, his head bowed, and I wondered if he was saying a silent prayer.

When the ambulance-men had gone and we had removed our barrier clothing, I turned to him.

'Whatever made you come and work in this place, before taking up your studies at the Theological College?' I enquired. 'You could have got a temporary job in an office or a factory, with shorter hours and more pay. You put up with the bad language, the lewd jokes, the drunks and the violence.'

'Why do you work here?' he asked in return.

'I don't really know. Do you?'

He paused before answering.

'Yes, I think I do. If I want to be a good shepherd, then I must know my flock.'

There was no answer that I could think of.

* * *

Throughout the year in every Accident and Emergency Department, the Grim Reaper does his work, and death in all its forms is close at hand. Perhaps the most traumatic incidents are the sudden deaths of people involved in road traffic accidents. On occasions, the victim's injuries were so bad that identification had to be made through their personal belongings. The younger age group were particularly at risk. One such driver, who was travelling at excessive speed along a country lane, collided with an oncoming tractor. He was decapitated, and when he was brought into Casualty, his head was in a plastic bag.

Motor cyclists were highly vulnerable, and most of those involved in road accidents were quite young. It was always a sad sight to view the victims when they arrived at the hospital dead, or badly injured. Taking anxious relatives to the Intensive Care Unit was a frequent duty, sometimes with the prior knowledge that the patient concerned had already died. The doctor or Sister on the ward had to break the news.

I was often asked to stay with a distressed relative in a side room if the person was alone. It was an emotive situation when a wife had to be told that the husband she had been married to for a great many years had died, or a husband had to be informed that his wife had been killed. At the request of the Sister in charge, some of these elderly people, without family and friends, were often driven home by me in the early hours of the morning, back to a house devoid of the warmth of companionship, and with a host of memories. If I could not summon help from a kindly neighbour, I would stay awhile and over a cup of tea listen while the bereaved relived the past and recounted old memories. The time would come, however, when no one would be at hand to offer comfort, and they would be alone in an empty house, in an empty room, with an empty chair.

One little old lady looked round her room at the photographs of her dead husband that surrounded her, and with the tears running down her cheeks asked: 'Why did he have to die at this time?'

Dear lady, I thought, there never is a right time to die.

Chapter 8

Creepers, Crawlies and Others

We live in deeds not years, in thoughts, not breaths,
In feelings, not in figures on a dial. We should
count time by heart-throbs. He most lives Who
thinks the most, feels the noblest, acts the best.

The usual Saturday night scene was in full swing as I pushed my way through the doors leading into the reception area of the Casualty Department. A group of people stood round the desk, waiting to be booked in. Debbie the receptionist was on the phone, and Jean, her companion, looked up from her work and gave me a wave. I glanced into the waiting room as I passed; it was obviously going to be a busy night, judging by the number of people inside.

Making my way to the staff room, which was in reality a glorified cupboard, I sorted out a white coat from the ones hanging on the hook behind the door. It must have been discarded by one of the doctors and I tried it on for size. It was always a compromise between a garment that enveloped me like a tent or one that was too small. Doctors seemed to be made differently from other people; they were either big and bulky or small and weedy. The coat I tried on, however, was near enough a fit, so I ignored the traces of blood on the sleeves and, after checking that there were no holes in the pockets, so that any blood specimens I had to carry to the Pathology Laboratory would not fall through, I was satisfied and ready for another weekend session. I opened the door and walked out to confront the city's suffering humanity.

'You're just the person I want,' said a voice behind me.

I turned round to find Sister bearing down on me.

'Take over the Consulting Room for me, and tell Nurse that she can go for her supper. When she comes back she can help with the patients in the cubicles.'

Taking over the Consulting Room meant acting as the casualty officer's receptionist. I had to collect the casualty cards from the desk for the patients suffering from minor injuries (or the walking wounded, as they were known to the staff) and then call them in to see the doctor when he was available. After the consultation, the card was handed back to me with the prescribed treatment written on it, such as medicine, dressings or X-rays, and then I recorded all the details in the record book before passing them on to the relevant nursing staff.

Filling in the treatment book and the X-ray book was keeping me busy in the corridor outside the Consulting Rooms. No desk or special facilities were available for this purpose, and I had to use the only flat surface I could find, which was a window ledge. I was quietly cursing under my breath when a male voice yelled in my ear:

'Have you seen my bloody organ?'

I swung round, startled by the voice, and took a pace backwards as I reacted to sour breath and a sweaty odour.

'I beg your pardon?'

'Have you seen my bloody organ?'

I was at a loss for words as I regarded the man who stood in front of me. I gave him one of my steely looks that I always imagined subdued any impertinence and commanded respect, but somehow this didn't seem to work with this client. He must have been in his mid sixties, and he had thinning grey hair. The dirty raincoat that he was wearing was far too large and it was wrapped round his body like a tent. It was held in the middle by a piece of string, as most of the buttons seemed to be missing. He was clutching in his hand a dirty brown trilby which was far too large for him, and when he put it on it rested on his ears. My silence seemed to enrage him, and he asked me for the third time: 'Well, have you seen my organ?'

I was at a loss to know how to answer him. I thought that I had better humour him.

'I'll get the doctor to take a look at it as soon as he's free. Give me your name and take a seat in the waiting room, please.'

He gave me a long withering look.

'You stupid sod!'

He stumbled to the reception desk and I dropped my pen and books on the window ledge and followed him. His voice bellowed out the question once again, and this time it was directed towards Debbie, who looked up from her desk.

'Have you seen my organ?'

I anticipated the worst. Was he going to tear open that dirty raincoat and reveal all? I came up behind him, ready to pounce, but to my surprise Debbie paused, turned round, picked up an object from behind her and handed it to the man.

'You left it on the counter Tom. We can't have our Larry Adler losing his mouth organ.'

That was my first introduction to Tom. The importance of that mouth organ to its owner did not occur to me until much later. Passing through the city's busy market place, I saw Tom standing in a shop doorway performing to the passing crowds. He was sucking and blowing on his instrument, and making weird noises. His old brown hat was on the ground with half a brick inside it to stop it blowing away. The music was all of Tom's making. There was no recognisable tune from his mouth organ, but when he played he seemed to be in another world. Alone with his fantasies, perhaps he was performing with some dream orchestra, and he was unaware of the ribald comments from the passing crowd.

Tom was a regular attendant at Casualty, and all the ambulance drivers knew him very well, through picking him up after he frequently collapsed in the street. These falls could not have been very serious as the staff would let him rest for an hour or so, give him a cup of tea, and tell him to go home. He would leave quietly clutching his mouth organ.

One busy evening, when an ambulance arrived with Tom inside, the Sister in charge gave a little groan when she saw him, and jokingly said:

'Oh Tom, we are very busy, can't you come back tomorrow?'

'Why yes, Sister,' he replied, and immediately jumped off the trolley. He made his way through the exit before anyone could stop him, ignoring the appeals of the staff to return.

Saturday night for Tom was also silver paper night, when he made his weekly visits to the Casualty Department to present to the duty receptionists a bag containing silver foil collected from milk bottle tops, chocolate wrappings and cigarette packets. Judging by the condition of the contents, Tom must have been scouring the gutters and delving in most of the city's dustbins. The foil was handed over with due ceremony, and received with profound thanks by the staff, who would congratulate him on his efforts. I never knew what became of the foil, but I strongly suspect that it finished up in the wastepaper basket. This foil-collecting was a legacy from the pre-National Health era, when the hospital depended on voluntary contributions and the efforts of the local population to raise funds. Collecting and selling large quantities of silver foil was one of the methods used, and Tom still remembered this from the past.

When Tom died, it was several weeks before the staff learnt of his passing. His familiar figure is no longer to be found in shop doorways in the city centre, but I do hope he managed to join that heavenly orchestra in the sky, sucking and blowing his mouth organ in time to the conducting angels.

* * *

Weekends in the Casualty Department always brought the same characters crowding into the waiting room, and I soon became acquainted with them all; perhaps more so than some of the regular staff, as they were on rotating shifts, while I worked the same hours each week. Some of the regulars, known as N.F.As, (no fixed abodes) never registered as patients but used the waiting room as a social centre. At night they inhabited the empty houses locally that were waiting to be pulled down to make room for the hospital's new wing. But in the meantime, the hospital waiting room beckoned, along with the possibility that some kind-hearted patient would perhaps buy them a cup of tea, or give them a cigarette. Many of these people were dirty, smelly and even flea-ridden, and it was not unusual for them to share their livestock with the staff. The extreme cases were known as the creepers and crawlers.

In the depth of Winter, the waiting room was a refuge for the homeless, and very often the police had to be called to remove the more violent types to avoid the whole area being turned into a hostel for the homeless. The staff were reluctant to take these measures; it was not a pleasant task to have these poor unfortunates evicted out into the streets on a cold Winter's night. But it had to be done, as the genuine patients, who included many children, would be subjected to a flow of bad language, the smell of foul, unwashed bodies, and harassing demands for money or cigarettes.

The cold weather also brought forth Steptoe, so named by the staff due to his appearance. I was first made aware of his presence when, on a cold Saturday night, I saw Tracey the staff nurse dash out through the doors of the main entrance and return shortly afterwards with a hospital blanket tucked under her arm.

'That was quick. What are you trying to do, Tracey, qualify for the Olympics?' I asked.

'It's a good job I was, with that thieving bugger about.' Tracey was not a person to mince her words.

'What do you mean?'

'Steptoe just walked out of here with this stuck up his jumper.' She indicated the blanket. 'He's the best blanket whipper in the business.'

Steptoe could not be described as having stepped out of a fashion magazine. He always wore an ex-army greatcoat both in Summer and Winter, grey and greasy in appearance. It had no buttons, and it was tied with the inevitable piece of string that was the hallmark of the dedicated wanderer. A cap that was too large for him was replaced according to the seasons by a Balaclava, and in extreme weather he tied pieces of cardboard round his ankles to form gaiters. At times rags were even added to his feet, either to keep them warm or to prevent water soaking through his shoes. He had an indescribable smell that not only preceded him but also lingered long after his departure. It was impossible to guess his age, as his unshaven face and matted hair acted as a disguise. I was never quite sure if he was very young or very old.

He usually visited Casualty on Saturday nights at about seven o'clock. This was after the local market stalls had closed, as evidenced by the large plastic bag he carried, full of over-ripe fruit and rotten vegetables he had begged or stolen from the stall holders. He was an expert scrounger examining the ashtrays in the waiting room for cigarette ends and checking the telephone kiosks for any loose coins. Even the newspapers left behind by patients and visitors joined the rest of his swag.

Blankets were a source of invaluable warmth to Steptoe. There were usually some left lying around in the waiting room by patients who had used them to keep warm while waiting for transport to take them home. It was then that Steptoe would strike. He would stuff one beneath his old army greatcoat and waddle away like some woman in the final stages of pregnancy.

The job of evicting Steptoe was always a duty that I was requested to do when the staff were busy, but it was difficult to keep him out. He knew the geography of the hospital so well that he would return a short time afterwards through another side entrance, and the procedure would start all over again. In the meantime, I had to make certain that there were no blankets lying around.

Many of the patients who had no fixed abode had evidently come from good backgrounds. It was obvious from their speech and mannerisms that they had not always followed their present mode of living, and were once clean and presentable. However, it was sad to see how degraded some of these people had become.

Old Joe, who was well known to the staff, was booked in one evening, quite ill with a chest infection. He was in a filthy state, and after being given a bath, he was admitted. It was the following night, when I had to take some X-rays to the ward, that I saw him again. It was change-over time, and the male charge nurse was handing over to the night sister at the bottom of Joe's bed.

'Are you feeling more comfortable now, Mr Bloggs?' he shouted to Joe, who was rather deaf. 'Don't worry, we will soon have you better again...' He turned to the night sister, and with a note of despair in his voice said, 'Watch him, the dirty bugger has shit himself twice today already.'

It was not only the men who comprised our group of creepers and crawlers. We also had some female members of this society, and amongst them, Helen was the senior member. She was, in her younger days, a Lady of the Night and, if she was to be believed, her services were in great demand during the war by the American forces stationed in the city. She was now old, homeless and an alcoholic. The Social Services had made great efforts to help her and had found her accommodation in various homes and hostels, but she refused to conform and never stayed in any of the places long. She always returned to her own mode of living on the streets. Her appearance was quite shocking: the bedraggled filthy clothes she was dressed in were never changed, the smell of stale urine enveloped her wherever she went, her matted hair hung in long strands and touched her shoulders. The grey blended with the darker roots and added to her unwashed look. Why she ever bothered to wear stockings puzzled mc, as they were so full of holes and ladders that if she ever took them off, which was doubtful, she would never get them back on again. Helen's shoes matched her hose, and I only recall her ever wearing one pair, which were black and down at heel. They were always noticeable as they were too large for her and always flopped about on her feet as she walked, as if they were going to drop off any minute. Helen would make her entrance in the afternoon just after the public houses had shut, and then her game of hide and seek with the staff would start as they tried to evict her. It was a game she nearly always won, as the staff eventually gave up trying after a time, owing to the pressure of work. The game would start again when I arrived on the scene in the evening. For some unknown reason, I had acquired the reputation of being able to get rid of unwanted vagrants from the waiting room (which was completely unjustified), and so her removal was left to me.

She could usually be found in Winter sitting in a wheelchair near the radiators to keep warm. In front of her, within convenient reach, would be one of the small occasional tables that were scattered around the room, the top littered with empty Guinness bottles. The contents had long been consumed before my arrival on the scene. The number of bottles varied from week to week according to how lucky she had been on her begging expedition over the lunch-hour. Used paper cups from the tea machine helped her imbibe in style, and the ashtray close at hand revealed the fact that she had managed to persuade some of the people in the waiting room to give her some cigarettes.

Helen always sat in a wheelchair. I think this was to evoke some sympathy from the other patients, who must have thought that she was waiting for treatment like themselves. There were periods when she could not hide her incontinence, however, and the result was a damp patch in the wheelchair and on the floor below her. From this position she would hold court, telling the people who were prepared to listen to her grand stories from the past, pausing only to beg a further cigarette and to re-check the Guinness bottles to make sure they were empty.

From this bundle of rags came a rich vibrant voice that would have been more at home in some drawing room, mingling with the sound of china teacups and the idle conversations of middle class ladies. She had a great command of the English language, but when she was upset she burst forth into a stream of invective that left you in no doubt that she was no lady. But there were times, on some quiet evenings, when she sat in a blend of light and shadow that seemed to enrich her face with a warm glow, and it was possible to glimpse the ghost of vanished beauty. Perhaps some of the grand stories she told were true, but now the past was her concern, and her future was in the hands of the Social Services. For the present, I had to turn her out on to the streets.

'Come along, Helen, it's time you were moving.'

'Hello, doctor, I'm having a bit of a rest.'

'I'm not a doctor.' She knew very well that I wasn't. 'Let's have you. You know that you can't stay here all night.'

'It's my legs, I can't walk.'

'Don't worry, I'll push you.'

With that I would grab the wheelchair and start to push her to the door, but not before she had gathered all her empty Guinness bottles into a large canvas bag she always carried. These returned empties represented hard cash towards her first drink later on that night. Once outside, Helen would step out of the chair, leaving a wet seat and a smell of urine behind.

'Don't come back, Helen, I've got to clean up all your mess.'

'You bloody fascist.'

I was always the bloody fascist to Helen, and I felt like one when I had to turn her out. To her I was the lowest form of humanity and perhaps she was right. I would watch her as she turned the corner out of sight, then I would re-enter the Department and walk along the corridor that led to the staff entrance, and wait. After a few minutes the outside door would slowly open, and after a brief pause Helen would step inside, blinking in the darkness before she became aware of my presence. I would slowly lift my arm when she saw me, and without speaking, point to the exit. Her reaction was always the same.

'You bloody fascist.'

The game would start all over again in a few hours' time when the pub closed, but in the meantime a mop and bucket were needed to clean up the mess. I could guess who would be asked to do it.

* * *

Almost all large hospitals have a file of names and sometimes photographs for quick and easy reference to identify the strange breed of patients known as Hospital Hoppers. While most people want to stay out of hospitals, there are a certain few who spend their lives trying to get into them, and when they are identified their names are circulated to most regional hospitals, as some of these people are known to operate over a large area of the British Isles.

Our Hospital Hoppers came in all shapes and sizes, and ranged from the very young to the very old. They were aware of the admission procedures at most hospitals, and could describe the symptoms of many illnesses and diseases with uncanny accuracy, which often mislead a busy casualty doctor into thinking he or she was treating a very sick patient. It was not always possible to probe into a patient's background and their stories had to be taken at face value when they reported to the Accident and Emergency Department. They usually told some plausible story about being a stranger in the city and having no doctor, or that they were on holiday, or just passing through, and it was impossible to distinguish them from the other patients from their mode of dress, unlike some of the down and out fraternity, who also reported sick on occasions to spend a few days in the warmth of the hospital. It might be some time afterwards before doubts arose in the minds of the hospital staff, after they had exhausted all known tests to find out what was wrong. But unfortunately by then, they had wasted the time of all types of professional staff, as well as occupying a bed on a ward that could have been allocated to a genuine patient.

Hospital Hoppers are very devious people. They know by an exchange of information which type of hospital has the most sympathetic staff, where the best food is served, and they also pick the units to suit their needs, ones that specialise in the illnesses they can describe. Our Accident and Emergency Department had its share of these people. Some lived locally, and although they were apt to change their names and give different addresses, some became well known to the staff. Even so, they had to be checked as a precaution if they turned up, just in case their illnesses were genuine. Sadly, it was a situation that had to be accepted, but was never condoned.

* * *

The Casualty waiting room was the Mecca for all sorts of strange people who required no medical attention. For some it was a convenient place to meet friends; some just turned up out of interest to watch all the activities of the staff and patients. The automatic drinks machine catered for casual callers at night when the pubs and cafes were closed, and the hospital toilets were in great demand by people passing.

Whenever there was any action taking place in the department, the Peeper was usually on the scene. He was a young man in his early twenties when I first got to know him, always well dressed in a conventional suit, a white shirt and tie. He would stand at the junction where the corridor and waiting room joined the reception area, and he monitored the incoming patients as they were booked in. This stream of humanity always fascinated him. He was never a nuisance apart from getting in the way occasionally, and it was pointless trying to get rid of him. Both the porters and nurses tried to move him on, but he would return after a time and take up his old position again, and they would finally give up. So he became part of the departmental furniture, and no one bothered him. The Casualty Department was a glimpse of the outside world to the Peeper, because he was deaf and dumb, frustrated by a lack of communication. Surrounded by activity, he seemed to enjoy watching all the things that were going on. When I arrived on the scene, he would give me a thumbs-up sign and make a little grunting noise; that was my greeting for the night. At ten o'clock precisely, his mother would walk into the department, tap him on the shoulder and, with a toss of her head, indicate the door, and he would meekly follow her outside. That would be the last I would see of him for that night.

But even the Peeper would draw the line at mixing with some of the Saturday night crowd. I had parked my car one evening, and just as I approached the main doors, Danny, the shift leader in charge of the porters, stood outside.

'Don't come in this way, Walter, use the ambulance bay.'

'What's wrong, Danny?'

The answer came as if on cue. A shower of glass fell at our feet as an object came flying through the window from inside the waiting room, and landed on the concrete apron nearby.

'What the hell is happening in there?'

'Brown and Brady are in there smashing up the waiting room.'

'Oh God, not that pair again. Have you sent for the police?'

'They're on the way.' He paused. 'Don't for Heaven's sake go in, the mood they're in, they could kill you.'

Being a natural-born coward, I had no intention of going in. The Brown-Brady combination was well known to the Casualty staff. They were regular attenders at the hospital, and their favourite tipple was a drink they called Red Biddy, a mixture of cheap red wine and methylated spirits, which didn't help to cement good relations with their fellow men. They became very violent at times when their requests, or rather their demands, to see a doctor were not immediately dealt with, and they were told to wait their turn. They were homeless because no institution would accept them owing to the trouble they caused, and the only time they had slept under a roof was when they were sent to prison by the local magistrates for breach of the peace. They had a habit of smashing shop windows in the city centre, and damaging public houses that had refused to serve them. Their relationship with the hospital stemmed back over a long period due to the injuries they sustained through their drunken brawls, and usually when they had been pieced together they showed some pangs of remorse and, in a way, some appreciation for the efforts of the staff who had treated them. But for some unknown reason tonight it was different.

I made my way through the ambulance bay and passed along the corridor towards the waiting room. The patients had already been evacuated to another area for their own safety while the fracas continued. I could hear the sound of banging noises and breaking glass as I got closer to the point where the porters stood sealing off the area.

'Can't we stop them?' I asked one of the porters.

'The nursing officer told us to wait for the police. He doesn't want any of the staff to get hurt.'

On reflection, it was sound advice. Attacks on hospital staff were on the increase. Glass windows could be replaced, but medical and nursing staff were too valuable to risk.

Twenty minutes later, the Brown and Brady duo were being bundled into the back of a police van, handcuffed and still struggling. As I surveyed the scene that they had left behind, I found it hard to believe that these two small figures had caused so much damage. The waiting room was a shambles; overturned chairs and tables littered the place, and glass from smashed windows covered the floor. The tax-payers were going to have to pay for the damage again, as the culprits had no money. I turned to Danny, the shift leader, who had now joined us.

'What made them go berserk?'

'You see that?' he asked, pointing to the drinks machine.

'Yes.'

'Well, they didn't like the taste of the tea.'

He turned away to start sweeping the waiting room floor, and then as a parting shot he went on:

'They said they were saving the patients from a fate worse than death.'

Well, if you ask a silly question ...

* * *

Sometimes, owing to climatic conditions, the Casualty Department had a spate of N.F.As of both sexes, and most of them were regulars and known to the staff. Some complained of all manner of illnesses, and booked themselves in to see a doctor, perhaps in the hope of spending a few days in a clean bed and having regular meals. Some certainly looked as if they needed medical treatment, and it was difficult to determine who was genuine; but every patient was examined irrespectively. The hospital had a Social Services Officer who was available during the day, and offered as much help as possible, but the N.F.As' mode of living never seemed to change, it was a way of life that they accepted. Arrangements were made to find some of them accommodation, and they were given new clothes and cash handouts, but sadly they soon returned to their old ways.

Holiday times brought a lot of down-and-outs into the hospital. Perhaps these forlorn people had a yearning for some human compassion during a period when family unity was at its strongest.

It was Easter Sunday when Mary the staff nurse pushed a casualty card into my hand. 'Get this patient for me, will you Walter – he's just in the waiting room in a wheelchair. He has a foot injury.'

'Yes, Staff.'

It was then I met Paddy Murphy. After calling out his name and receiving an answer, I discovered him in his wheelchair, isolated from the rest of the patients. I think he must have been one of the dirtiest men I have ever seen, and the bodily odours emanating from him made me realise why he sat apart from the other people in the room. The clothes he was wearing were in rags, and they were stained and greasy. His dirty face had not been touched with water for a long time, and the stubble on his chin varied in colour from a dirty grey to a matted brown shade. He had no hat to cover his long hair, and he didn't appear to have any worldly goods. If he did, he must have carried them on his person. I reached for the handle of the wheelchair and started pushing it from the rear, and then I saw the fleas on the back of his neck above the collar of his coat.

After working in the department for a long time, I should have been used to the sight of these little creatures, but I wasn't, and I always treated them with the greatest of respect. I get an immediate itch that stays with me, and I instinctively want to scratch when I see them.

Holding the wheelchair at arms length, I pushed the patient into the consulting room area, where Mary was waiting. As she came forward, I pointed to the patient from behind and started scratching my head, underneath my arms, and across my body, making faces at the same time. Mary watched me with a puzzled look on her face.

'What the hell's the matter with you?' she asked. 'If you are going to have a nervous breakdown, go and do it somewhere else, we are too busy to bother about you.'

With that, she wheeled Paddy Murphy into the doctor's room, but not for long. After about two minutes she came out again and swept past me, still pushing Paddy in the wheelchair, and then she left him in a small alcove at the end of the corridor.

'What's the matter, Mary?' I asked.

'The doctor won't see him until he's had his foot washed.'

'The best of British luck to you. That patient has more fleas on him than you have hairs on your head.'

She looked directly at me. 'I wasn't thinking of doing it myself,' she said.

'Who's going to do it then?'

Mary didn't answer but gazed at me with those big brown Irish eyes of hers, and then she wrinkled her nose and smiled. She had a way with her that few people could resist, and she used her charm to work wonders. I suddenly realised what her silence indicated.

'Oh, no,' I said. 'Not me ... never.'

'Not even for suffering humanity?'

'No ... no ... NO!'

'I knew you would,' she said, and with another wrinkle of her nose and a little smile, she left me standing in the corridor.

It was some time later when I approached Paddy. I was now attired in barrier clothing, covered by a green theatre gown with a plastic apron top, and with the added protection of gloves, headgear, a face mast and overshoes. I felt like some surgeon ready to operate. Nearby was a bowl of warm water, a bottle of antiseptic and some dressings. I knelt down besides Paddy's wheelchair.

'Which is your bad foot, Paddy?' I asked.

'It's my right foot, Sir. Can you let me have a cigarette?'

'You can't smoke here.'

To remove his shoe I had to remove the string that was threaded through the first two eyelets. His foot was very swollen, and as I held his ankle, I saw Paddy wince with pain when I removed it. His sock beneath was wet and sticky, and the smell was terrible. Before proceeding any further, I rolled his trouser leg up to below his knee, and his exposed skin was black with dirt. Now it was time to remove his sock, and when I tried to peel it off, it was rotten from the sweat and dirt that clung to it. As I rolled it down to his ankle, I could feel the moisture oozing out at my touch, in spite of the gloves that I was wearing. Trying to be as gentle as possible, I pulled the sock round the ball of his foot to avoid causing him pain, and with a final tug I completed the operation and dropped it on the floor. To my surprise, there was a dressing on the foot itself, and although it was as filthy as the sock, it had obviously been put on by someone with nursing experience.

'Who put the dressing on your foot, Paddy?'

'Dressing, what do you mean?'

'The bandage?'

'That was done before I left prison.'

'Prison? How long ago was that?'

'I can't remember. Four or five weeks.'

'And you haven't had it changed?'

'No. I had a letter to bring to the hospital but I lost it. I thought I'd try to get some money from the Social Security before I came to see a doctor.'

'Where have you been living since then?'

'Anywhere I can, but mostly I've been dossing in empty houses round the corner.'

I snipped the edges of the dirty plaster that was used to hold the bandage and gently started to unroll the dressing. As I unwound it towards the toes I saw it was stuck by a mass of discharge to the foot itself. As I eased it, the flesh beneath it seemed to be rotten and clinging to it was a piece of lint. The smell was even worse now as the bandage joined the shoe and sock on the floor.

As I put Paddy's foot in the bowl, the water immediately changed colour and the lint eased a little from the skin. I could now see more clearly the suppurating mass of flesh that should have been Paddy's right toes, as I removed the lint. His foot seemed to be rotting away, and I felt quite sick at the sight of it. I also felt a deep anger. How could a human being in a civilised society neglect himself like this; or was society neglecting the Paddys of this world?

I changed the water in the bowl at least five times, and with the antiseptic from the bottle the foot had now taken on a grey appearance, but the toes were still black and discharging. My knees and back ached from kneeling in the small alcove, and I started drying Paddy's foot by lightly pressing on an absorbent dressing, trying not to cause him pain.

'Haven't you finished yet?' Mary's voice came from behind me. 'The doctor's waiting to see the patient. It's taking you a long time.'

'Look for yourself, Staff Nurse, you'll see the reason why.'

She bent over to look at the foot, and gazed at it in silence for a few seconds. She could see the black line on Paddy's leg to where I had washed it, and I saw her face change at the sight of his toes and the weeping black flesh. The smell permeated through my mask, and I could imagine the effect that it was having on Mary.

'Holy Mother of God,' she whispered. 'I never realised it was so bad. I thought he had a bone injury.'

I was still on my knees drying the foot. Mary watched me from behind. After a while, she spoke.

'You do know what day it is today?'

'I'm not likely to forget, it's Sunday.'

'It's Easter Sunday.'

'Well I'm sorry, I haven't brought you an Easter egg.'

'I was at Church over Easter, and the Priest always washes the feet of some of the congregation to symbolise the actions of Jesus. Seeing you reminded me of it.

‘Well I hope their feet were cleaner than Paddy’s’

I stood up and stretched my aching back, Mary came forward and pulled the wheelchair into the corridor. ‘I’ll take over now,’ she said, and started pushing Paddy towards the doctor’s room. She stopped briefly and looked back over her shoulder.

‘What a saint you are,’ she said.

The saint developed a sudden itch under his barrier clothing as he stood wondering what to do with one rotten sock and an old shoe with a hole in it.

One thing for sure; he would give supper a miss that night.

* * *

The police car pulled up outside the entrance and blocked the access, allowing only limited passage for people to squeeze by. I stood near the reception desk and was about to remonstrate with the driver when the young constable responsible for the obstruction put his head round the door and grinned.

‘Where do you want it then?’ he asked.

‘Where do I want what?’ I replied.

‘I’ve got their gear here.’

‘Whose gear?’

‘Dot and Carry’s.’

I looked across the counter to Jo the receptionist, and wondered if she was more enlightened than I was. To my surprise, she seemed to know what the poor demented officer of the law was talking about.

‘Is there much?’ she asked.

‘My back seat’s full of their stuff, it’s a wonder you can’t smell it.’

Jo looked over at me. ‘Would you give him a hand,

Walter? Put all of it in the passage for the time being, I don't want it this side of the counter.'

Somewhat perplexed, I followed the policeman outside, and as he unlocked the rear door of his car I could see the "stuff" he'd been referring to. It was piled in the back and almost obscured the rear window. There were blackened pots and pans, dirty looking blankets tied with string, bundles and parcels of all shapes and sizes, plastic bags, canvas bags, bottles containing water, a bowl and bucket and incredibly a bowler hat lying on top of the heap. The whole of the contents emitted a sour smell, and I could well understand why the police constable was anxious to get rid of his load.

'Where did you get this lot from?' I asked.

'Oh, from a village about eight miles away. We had a message to say that Dot had been brought in to Casualty suffering from an arm injury after being hit by a passing car. I gather it's not too serious, but I was told to bring her belongings.'

Not having the faintest idea who Dot was, I gave a hand to unload the police car and we piled them along the corridor wall to the dismay of the Sister in charge, who was not very pleased at the sight. The young constable, however, was in a lighter mood. He borrowed the air freshener spray from behind the reception desk and went to work with it on the rear seat. Then, satisfied with his lavender smelling car, he got in and lowered the window.

'Thanks for your help, they're all yours now. You won't see me again.' He waved and drove off.

The story of Dot and Carry unfolded over the next hour. They were unique personalities of the tramp world. Dot was a woman in her late forties with very short straight hair, a wrinkled weather-beaten face, brick red in colour, and on the two occasions that I met het she was wearing a pair of men's boots and trousers that had seen better days. She was a dominant woman, powerful in personality, and the complete opposite to the man in her life, Carry, her husband or partner. He was the quiet type, always at her elbow, obeying her every command without question, like a trained dog.

They both travelled along the highways and byways of England and Wales with all their goods and chattels. They were known to most of the local police forces as they crossed over the county boundaries, and they were regarded with a kindly eye, as they caused no trouble. The procedures involved in moving their belongings were somewhat unusual, hence their names Dot and Carry. They were so burdened by their worldly goods, it was impossible to carry them all at once, so they adopted the method of moving them in relays. They would transport their belongings a few hundred yards along the road, leave them and return for another load until all their goods had been moved. They would then repeat this procedure, and work their way slowly across the countryside until they found a convenient spot to spend the night. Various authorities were concerned about their welfare, but offers of help were ignored. Dot maintained her stubborn independence and Carry followed blindly in her footsteps.

An hour and a half later, I saw Dot stalk out of the Fracture Clinic, her lower right arm encased in plaster. She was followed by the Sister in charge.

'We'll find you somewhere to stay so we can check that arm,' Sister said. 'You can't go yet.'

'You're not keeping us in here,' came the reply. 'Where's our luggage? We want to be taken back to where we came from. I didn't ask to be brought here.'

I withdrew tactfully from the scene when Dot demanded an ambulance to transport her back, and Sister told her she couldn't have one. The exchange developed into a rather heated argument.

It was some time later when Jo the receptionist found me helping the porters.

'Sorry to trouble you again, Walter, but could you give Dot and Carry a hand with their goods? They're on the move again.'

I went along the corridor, picked up some of their bundles and made my way to the door. The same police car stood waiting with its rear door open, and the same young fresh-faced constable stood beside it.

'I thought you had said goodbye to us,' I remarked.

A look of disgust came over his face.

'Another ten minutes and I would have been off duty. Now look what I've let myself in for.'

We loaded all the goods into the back of the car, and Carry was buried underneath them somewhere, while Dot went and sat in front with the driver, who was looking far from pleased. He started the engine and turned to me.

'Have we got everything?' he enquired.

'No, wait a second, there is one other item.'

I dashed inside and handed it to him. 'I think you'll need it,' I said as I handed him the air freshener.

* * *

It was a warm Summer evening and the waiting room was full of people all suffering from seasonal complaints that could be associated with the weather. There were incidents of children falling from trees, traffic accidents, mainly involving weekend drivers, bone injuries, and twisted limbs due to sporting activities; not to mention various forms of illnesses that could be treated by the patients' own GPs at a later date.

All the porters were busy and I was standing in the passage cleaning a trolley when Cynthia the staff nurse stopped and stared down the corridor towards the entrance with an enquiring look on her face. She turned to me.

'Who's that man?' she asked. 'He's behaving very strangely and jumping up and down like a scalded cat.'

I turned round and saw the approaching figure hopping towards us.

'Oh, that's Sam, he's one of our regulars.'

'What does he want?'

'You'll soon find out,' I replied.

Sam came hopping along on one foot and then the other, and seeing us watching him, he turned and made his way in our direction.

'I know what he's going to say,' I said.

'What's that?' Cynthia asked.

'He can't piss.'

'I'm surprised at you Walter,' she said. 'That's not your usual language.'

Sam came right up to us and clung to the wall and stood on one leg.

'Oh ... I can't piss ... I can't piss ...' were the first words he uttered.

'It's his usual retention problem.' I turned to Cynthia. 'Look after him, I'll go and book him in. I know all his details, he's been in here several times over the last few months.'

Although it was a hot day, Sam was wearing the dirty raincoat that he used as a dressing gown, and underneath he was adorned in his underwear, which consisted of a heavy vest and woollen longjohns that had not been washed for a very long time, if the smell of urine that clung to them was any indication. Sam was elderly and unshaven. His thinning grey hair stood vertically on his head, creating a grotesque appearance. He always came at the most awkward times and his presence was heralded by the loud declaration: 'I can't piss ... I can't piss ...' as he hopped up and down on his legs.

Sam lived about half a mile away from the hospital and had to cross two main roads to reach the Casualty Department. His mode of dress always aroused great interest on the way, and he was at one time accompanied by the police. They wondered if they had a case of indecent exposure to deal with, as he wandered the streets clad only in his dirty raincoat, his longjohns and vest.

When the highest lady in the land was due to honour us by opening the new extension of the hospital, I was kindly invited to the ceremony, and as she was due to tour the Accident and Emergency Department, I waited in line with Sister Sue. I turned to Sue.

'I wonder what Her Majesty would say if Sam came in now shouting, "I can't piss ... I can't piss ...".'

'I don't know what the Queen would say,' said Sue. 'But I know what her husband would answer.'

'What's that?'

'Piss off!'

Chapter 9

The Face of Violence

They are not long, the weeping and the laughter.
Love and desire and hate: I think they have no portion in us after We pass the gate.

The city had two faces, one by day and one by night. As the hours lengthened and the twilight melted into darkness, the sinister face emerged. Violence was at hand throughout the day, but it was at night that I came face to face with it. The staff in every Accident and Emergency unit knew it in all its forms, and suffered from the effects of it, as attacks on hospital workers increased year by year. There was a period in the past when the general public held in high regard doctors, nurses, teachers, the Police and other professional bodies, and appreciated all the work they did for the community. But sadly, liberty for some means license for others to indulge in anti-social behaviour.

In the dark corners of the city, in the shop doorways, the car parks and the public toilets, there were always people lurking in the shadows to take advantage of the late night reveller returning home, or the worker finishing his shift. These were potential victims, usually good for a few pounds. Little old ladies and young girls were also easy prey for the muggers and bag-snatchers. The thieves responsible for such acts were blindly unaware of the deep mental scars their victims suffered afterwards.

Sexual deviants were also at risk, as the city had several underground toilets in my early days at the hospital, and these attracted certain types of male homosexuals. Occasionally they would be invaded by gangs of youths on what were known as "queer-bashing" raids. The occupants would be beaten up, and the offenders would be gone before any help could arrive. Although the police were aware of these attacks, there were very few complaints from the victims, as they wanted no publicity regarding their sexual habits. Some were prominent people in the public eye, and they always fabricated some story to explain their injuries. The most popular reasons given were walking into doors, falling over kerbstones and falling down stairs. But I would assume by the location of the injuries that the stairs must have reared up and hit them.

Joe was a victim of the queer-bashing fraternity and he was brought to the hospital by the Police, who had found him in a dazed condition outside one of the more notorious underground toilets just after midnight. He was suffering from severe cuts and bruises on his face. Judging by the imprints on his clothes, he had also been trampled on while he was on the ground. In spite of his injuries, he insisted that he wanted to go home, but Sister was concerned about his condition and ignoring his protests, she finally persuaded him to stay. She asked me to undress him, so I took him to a side cubicle to perform the task, although I could sense his reluctance.

Poor Joe was a pathetic figure. He must have been in his late fifties or even older – it was hard to tell. He was wearing a film of make-up which consisted of lipstick that was now smeared round his mouth, and rouge on his cheeks which made his face look like an over-ripe apple. When I removed his coat I discovered that he was wearing a black wig, the type that was on sale at any joke shop and was popular during the Beatles era. It was a bad fit, and the edges of his whiskery grey hair showed below it.

It was when I took off his shoes that I realised his other dress was somewhat unconventional. I could not remove his socks, and the mystery was solved when I removed his trousers and exposed the rest of his nether garments. He was wearing a brown pair of ladies' bloomers, the type with elasticated legs. Protruding through the bottom of these were four suspenders hooked on to a pair of very thick black stockings that I had at first mistaken for socks. Unbuttoning his shirt, I caught a glimpse of the ladies' vest he was wearing, which did not quite cover the dirty-looking laced corset that was wrapped round his body. I decided to investigate no further, so I covered Joe with a blanket and went to find Sister, who could advise me how to proceed.

She was in her office in conversation with a detective from the Vice Squad who had brought Joe to the hospital. She looked up as I entered.

'Is Joe undressed?' she asked.

'As far as possible, Sister, but he's wearing some funny garments. I wouldn't remove them all until I had words with you.'

The detective looked up.

'Don't tell me he's still wearing those bloody brown bloomers?'

'I'm afraid so. How did you know?'

'We had him inside a few weeks ago, and he was wearing them when we searched him. I don't mind dealing with queers, but I get all the ugly buggers. It would be nice to have a change.'

'I'll let you know when we have a suitable model in stock,' I replied.

The ladies of the night, who followed the oldest profession, accepted the fact that violence was always an occupational hazard. The threat came not only from their clients but also from their so-called protectors. It was not uncommon on some nights to see a large American car draw up to the entrance of Casualty where the driver, a large West Indian, would deliver one of his many ladies for treatment. He was a very big man, well over six feet tall, and dressed in a brightly coloured suit. He also wore a wide-brimmed circular hat, a type of stetson like the ones worn by John Wayne in the cowboy films of that era.

Known as Flash Harry to the porters, he was reputed to have a string of girls working for him in the red light area of the city. It was said that he controlled them by withholding the drugs he supplied to them, and using his fists if that didn't work. It was at a later date that these suspicions were confirmed when he was not seen for some time, and the local newspaper revealed that he had been sentenced to four years in gaol for living off immoral earnings. I hardly think he left many broken hears behind with his departure. But it simply meant that a vacancy had been created for someone to take his place.

In spite of the injuries that some of the prostitutes suffered, they rarely made any official complaints against the person responsible. It may have been from fear, or reluctance to put their profession in jeopardy by dealing with the police. Some of the more seriously injured victims were interviewed by police officers who knew who the assailants were, but they were frustrated in their efforts to bring charges by the code of silence that existed.

Among the many prostitutes walking the city's streets was a frequent patient in the Casualty Department, Marlene. Apart from her occasional habit of "walking into doors, and falling down stairs", she was at times found collapsed in the street, suffering from either an over-indulgence of alcohol or drugs. She was in her mid-thirties but looked much older. She had been plying her trade since she was a teenager, and some of the long-serving members of the Casualty staff had known her and treated her over a long period. They had established a good rapport with her.

Marlene was always dressed in the same type of clothing when I saw her – a very short skirt and a top with a plunging neckline. It was like a uniform that symbolised her profession. She must have been very attractive when she was younger, but the combination of drink, drugs and her mode of living had taken its toll over the years. Her relationship with the staff was always on a personal basis, and any dialogue usually ended with Marlene having the last word.

'What's happened to you this time, Marlene? Did you trip over a kerbstone or fall down the stairs?' someone would ask.

'No, I was raped by a sex maniac from the Casualty Department.'

Like the rest of her sisters, she never complained to the police, even when she came for treatment for a slashed cheek that needed stitching, which had obviously been done with a knife or razor. She insisted that she had walked into a glass door and shattered it. This was a new story for Marlene, and even though she was questioned by the police, who suspected that her minder had committed the offence, she stuck to her story.

On another occasion when she came in after being assaulted, Sister Sue was on duty. She gave a sigh when she saw Marlene.

'Oh not again, Marlene, this is the second time you've been in this month.'

'No, Sister, it's the third time. I had a check-up in your VD Clinic.'

Sue, never a lady to mince her words, gave another sigh and shook her head.

'You must be costing the National Health Service a fortune. Why don't you piss off to London and give us a rest. You could earn more money there.'

'I'm doing fine here,' Marlene answered. 'I can earn more money in a day than you can earn in a month.'

'If that thing between your legs is as big as your mouth, I'm not surprised,' said Sue, and she walked away before Marlene could answer.

There were many young girls and women like Marlene. Some boasted openly about their high earnings, but kept quiet about their ongoing costs, such as the men who lived off their bodies and drove around in high-powered cars and the landlords who wanted their share of the income in the form of extortionate rents for the rooms they hired out so the girls could entertain their clients. But above all, they never realised what the constant abuse of their bodies by sex, drink and drugs really cost them, a cost that could not be reckoned in terms of money.

* * *

I was always puzzled by the fact that experts who offer advice are usually remote from the situations they claim to be knowledgeable about. One such person, writing in a medical journal, stated that much of the violence suffered by the staff in Accident and Emergency Departments was of their own making because they did not understand the needs of this particular type of patient. By talking to them, and finding the reasons for their anger, most of these situations could be resolved peacefully, the writer claimed.

Well, one thing's for sure, that writer had never worked in a busy Casualty Department. Offering tea and sympathy to patients high on drugs, or whispering sweet words in the ears of a raving mad drunk who is ready to take on the rest of the world, is not, I'm afraid, going to help the staff avoid getting punched, kicked or bitten in the course of their duties.

Included in this category was Kevin, a patient I came to

know very well over the years. My first introduction to him was when he was brought in by the police along with one of his victims. Apparently Kevin was going through a phase at that time of throwing himself at cars, not underneath them, but bouncing off their bonnets. This greatly upset the drivers, and in this particular incident the driver was a lady who was so upset she too was brought to the hospital.

There was no doubt that Kevin needed medical help, but his actions did not endear him to the staff on his frequent visits. Kevin hated all the portering staff, and would think nothing of throwing a punch at any unsuspecting new member who approached him offering help. Sympathy from the staff was regarded by him as weakness, and on occasions they would yield to his subtle blackmail when he demanded cups of tea or cigarettes, just to keep him quiet. His appearance in the department would occupy the attention of up to three porters for as long as the staff would tolerate him before calling the police, who would then come and remove him.

From jumping into the front of cars he then progressed to jumping into the local canal, but always making sure the police knew his intentions, so that they could come and rescue him. Again, he was not the most popular person when he dragged a rescuing officer in with him. He reached the peak of his career when he committed several acts of arson. He was later convicted for these crimes and sent to a different type of hospital, a very secure one for the criminally insane. Life in Casualty was more peaceful after his departure.

Enclosed in the city boundary was a high security prison, and this establishment housed many notorious characters who were serving long sentences for their crimes. Through overcrowding and a nothing-to-lose attitude by some of the long term inmates, the gaol was a hotbed of violence. On many occasions, prisoners were rushed into Casualty suffering from stab wounds from implements that were made surreptitiously, and secreted away by some inmates, then used to settle old scores when the opportunity arose. Cases of patients suffering from severe burns and scalds from feuds that arose in the prison kitchens had to receive urgent treatment in the Burns Unit. Most of these patients were confined to side rooms in the hospital and guarded by the prison officers that accompanied them. In spite of all the security precautions, however, one prisoner did manage to escape, wearing a pair of hospital pyjamas. Making the excuse that he wanted to go to the toilet, he managed to squeeze through a small window about eighteen inches square and drop nearly twenty feet to the garden below. In a short time the hospital was surrounded by police, who combed the whole area without success. The nursing staff, especially those working at night, went about their duties afterwards with a deep sense of apprehension, convinced that the escaped convict was hiding in some dark recess in the hospital. The portering staff tried to allay their fears by escorting them when they had to leave their wards for a meal break. And so the local gaol lost a prisoner, and the National Health Service a pair of pyjamas.

* * *

It was the year in 1981 of the long hot Summer and people sweltered under the humid heat that seemed to go on for ever. In the slums and ghettoes of the large cities to the north and south, there were rumblings of discontent amongst the ethnic minorities and some of the white population. As the hot weather continued, the rumblings turned into riots, and as the riots spread, the mobs took over. Our Accident and Emergency Department was aware of this situation, and there was a close liaison between the hospital, the police and the emergency services, as there were fears that the trouble would spread in a copy-cat manner. It did. When it started, it was in a minor way on a Friday night, with groups of people gathering in the streets, cars being pelted with stones as they passed, and some windows being broken. But on Saturday night it reached a climax. I was helping Ron, the night clerk, on the reception desk. For a weekend it had been comparatively quiet so far, and it was a telephone call to the Sister in charge that changed the whole tempo of the department. She broke the news to Ron.

'The police have just phoned to say that there has been an outbreak of rioting near the city centre, and we can expect some casualties, so stand by. I'll alert the nursing officer.'

It was not long before the first ambulance arrived, carrying two police officers suffering from head injuries caused by flying stones.

'What's happening in our big city?' I asked Mike the ambulance-man.

'The whole place is likely to go up in flames,' he said. 'The mob has started to loot some of the city centre shops. The white yobs have got in on the act now, it's not just a race riot. The mobs are stealing anything they can lay their hands on and the police are having difficulty in containing them. They're sending for reinforcements.'

From a quiet beginning the momentum increased and a constant stream of patients kept us busy filling in casualty cards with all the relevant personal details. In most cases, in the section marked "illness or injury", the word "assault" was added.

Mike returned again, this time with a long-haired youth who looked rather the worse for wear. He was badly bruised around the face, and was protesting loudly as he entered. I took his details and wrote the word "assault" in the appropriate section of the card.

'You can f.....g alter that,' he said, stabbing his finger

through the opening in the glass screen and pointing to the word.

'What are you on about?' I queried.

'I want that altered to "assault by police".'

'I'm sorry, I can't do that.'

'It's my bleeding card.'

'This card belongs to the hospital, not to you.'

'Look what those bastards did to me,' he went on, pointing to his face. 'I want you to report the fact.'

'If you have any complaints relating to the conduct of the police, you must make them yourself. We are here to tend your injuries.'

'I'm going to write to my MP about this, he'll have your guts for garters. What's your name...?'

'Why don't you shut your bloody big gob and belt up,' said Mike the ambulance-man, who had now appeared on the scene, and with that he took the casualty card from my hand and led the still protesting youth away.

The casualty staff had now been reinforced by doctors and nurses from the wards, and some staff on the on-call list. The number of patients had increased from both sides of the battle lines. Most of the police casualties were suffering from head injuries caused by flying stones, and some of the rioters, who had made their own way to the hospital, had badly lacerated hands, presumably caused by breaking shop windows. The waiting room was now awash with police, patients and relatives, all demanding instant treatment and information. Some of the coloured members of the community were complaining about the racist staff who were giving priority treatment to the white patients, while the police were busy keeping a group of white youths apart from some West Indians that they wanted to eliminate, claiming they were responsible for their injuries.

It was four o'clock in the morning before the rioting died

down. The police, with the help of some neighbouring forces, managed to contain the mobs. The damage was widespread throughout the city centre: shops had been looted, cars overturned, houses and factories damaged. Police cars and ambulances were prime targets, and help for some of the victims who lived in the area taken over by the rioters was delayed. It was only through the dedication of the men and women of the two services that they managed to stem the flood of violence.

Mike, the ambulance-man, was still bringing patients in as I was leaving.

'Do you get danger money on your job, Mike?' I asked.

'Piss off home,' he replied.

As I made my way along the corridor to get my coat, the youth who had been complaining about police brutality was lying on a trolley waiting for an X-ray.

'Do you still want to complain about the police?' I asked.

'Too bloody true,' came the reply.

I pushed him further along the corridor and put him by the side of a young police constable, a victim of the mob violence, whom I had booked in previously, and whose head was now covered in bandages.

'This man wants to complain about police brutality,' I said. 'And he wants to talk to a policeman.' I turned to the youth. 'This patient is a policeman, and he didn't get his injuries through police brutality.'

The young constable looked up from his pillow and gazed at the youth.

'He'll find out what police brutality really means if he doesn't shut his bloody mouth,' he said.

The youth made no reply, and I thought it prudent to push him back to his original place along the corridor.

Sunday night brought some spasmodic fighting that was soon brought under control by the police, and although the staff in Casualty were on the alert for any emergency, the situation eased and finally tapered off in the following week. The cost of the damage was considerable, and once again the money came from the public purse and the insurance companies. The local and national newspapers had a field day with banner headlines about race riots. But to me it just seemed to have been a great opportunity for the malcontents of all races to challenge the established authority by rioting and looting.

* * *

Then there was the violence of a different kind.

The queue waiting to go to the X-ray Department was lengthening, and I pulled the first trolley out of line to take the patient along the corridor. From the head of the vehicle I could see the dark hair of the young lady on the trolley spread over the white pillow. She made an effort to sit up and turn round.

'Aren't you going to say hello to me?' she said.

I paused and looked at her, and her face did look familiar; but it was some seconds before I realised who she was.

'I'm sorry, but you look different without your uniform,' I said.

WPC Anne Green was a regular visitor to the Casualty Department when she was on official business, but she looked quite different tonight in her civilian dress, and hardly one's idea of a policewoman. She looked so young as she lay on top of the trolley with a hospital blanket half-covering her blue dress, and with her left leg propped up on a pillow.

'Here you are, you're not on duty today, and you've been injured yourself. What have you done to your leg? Have you been living it up in our great city?'

'No, I've been living it down in the ladies' toilets, on observation duty.'

'Haven't the ladies been putting their pennies in the slots then?'

'No. There's been a spate of handbag snatching lately.'

I pondered on the crime statistics relating to ladies' toilets and failed to come up with a logical answer.

'You're joking, of course,' I said. 'How do you snatch handbags in ladies' toilets?'

'Well, they go inside, lock the door, put their handbags on the floor and sit down on the seat.'

'So what happens then?'

'Then some unscrupulous person comes along, puts her hand under the gap at the bottom of the door, snatches the handbag and runs away. The victims are caught at a disadvantage. It happened tonight, but unfortunately when I chased after the thief, I slipped and fell down the stairs, and hurt my leg. The thief got away and I ended up here.'

'You might say that they were all caught with their pants down,' I said. 'That's the reason why men have pockets in their trousers.'

'Don't be bloody cheeky,' Anne said.

Chapter 10

The Young Ones

Soft my child. I did not chide thee, Though my song might sound too hard; 'Tis thy mother sits besides thee, And her arms shall be thy guard.

It was a quiet Saturday night, and the evening sunshine had stretched the shadows in the hospital square. Two white-clad figures carrying tennis rackets walked slowly along the path in the direction of the Nurses' Home. I turned away from the window in the Casualty Department and moved along the corridor, glancing into the waiting room where a few patients with minor injuries were waiting to see a doctor. It was supper time and the casualty officer who had been on duty all day had taken advantage of this quiet period to go for a meal. As I waited I reflected on my forthcoming holiday in Scotland, and dreamed of long quiet walks in the hills, the smell of heather and the breeze blowing in my face. But my visions were short-lived, as Eric the ambulance-man pushed his way through the swing doors carrying a small boy in his arms.

'Is this trolley free?' he asked.

'Help yourself.'

The boy looked frightened as Eric placed him on the trolley. His dirty face and runny nose underlined the look of neglect about him. He was wearing shorts and his socks had slipped down to his ankles, showing the ingrained dirt on his legs. He must have been about eight or nine years old.

'Is the doctor about?' asked Eric.

'No, he's gone to dinner.'

'This young boy is an overdose. His father is booking him in.'

'What's he taken?' I asked.

'Anti-mating fluid for bitches.'

I looked at the young boy and wondered if it was a joke, but Eric was not the type to make jokes. He took his job very seriously.

'Have you brought him to the right place?'

'What do you mean?'

'You should have taken him to see a vet.'

'You've got enough bloody vets working here,' Eric replied.

It was a sick joke on my part, but one that I could not resist. The young patient would need priority treatment; the term overdose applied to any patient who had accidentally or deliberately swallowed any liquids or solids that could be a danger to their health, and a delay in treatment could have serious consequences. I reported the arrival of the young patient to Sister, who bleeped for a doctor.

The boy was wheeled into the children's treatment room and the staff nurse did all the preliminary observations of his condition ready for the doctor, while Sister checked the card index system that listed all the poisons and drugs, and any antidotes. These cards also described the resulting symptoms and the treatment required, and although there were many veterinary products listed, there was not a word about anti-mating fluid for bitches. Sister reported the lack of success to the doctor who had now arrived on the scene.

'Did you bring the bottle with you?' the doctor asked the small man standing in the background, who turned out to be the boy's father.

'No, I left it behind.'

'I told you to bring it,' said Eric. 'We could have checked the label.'

'There was no label on it,' said the father. 'But it was made by Bloggs Products for dogs.'

The doctor turned to Sister. 'Phone Guy's Hospital and see what they come up with.'

Guy's Hospital in London was the main information centre for toxic substances, and it was used by the provincial hospitals when their own poison files were incomplete. At Guy's, the register listed thousands of substances, many not in general use. The answer to our enquiry came back very quickly. Anti-Mating Fluid had its uses when applied to certain members of the canine family, but it was definitely not recommended as a drink for small boys. It could cause nausea, vomiting and other internal problems.

'How much did he drink?' asked the doctor.

'I don't know,' replied the father, 'but he should know.' And he pointed to his son.

The doctor tried again.

'How much did you drink, laddie?'

The boy looked round at the white-coated figures that surrounded him, a strand of matted hair fell over his forehead and his tongue flicked out to remove the drip that ran from his nose. Sister, with a look of disgust, reached behind her and handed the small patient a paper tissue, and the lad proceeded to wipe his nose while everyone waited.

'Listen,' the doctor went on. 'This is most important, and we are trying to help you. How much of the liquid did you swallow?'

The boy looked round and paused.

'I didn't swallow any of the bleeding stuff. It tasted 'orrible so I spat it out.'

The doctor sighed, Eric the ambulance-man pursed his lips, Sister remained silent, the staff nurse looked down at her feet to hide a smile and the boy's father shuffled further back into the corner of the room, trying to hide his embarrassment.

'Do his observations again in another hour,' the doctor

said. 'We may keep him in overnight to make sure he's alright. We'll see how he goes.' He left the room, followed by Sister and with Eric running at their heels.

The boy's father came out of his corner with a sheepish look on his face. 'Well, I didn't know, did I?' was all he could say.

'No,' I replied. 'You did the right thing, it's better to be safe than sorry.'

* * *

Children are absolutely unpredictable in their behaviour. From a very early age they do the most outrageous things as they start learning, which could lead to dire consequences. Babies begin exploring their small world when they start crawling, and it might be reasonable to hope that by the time they have reached the age of four or five they will be aware of some of the dangers that surround them. But it's not always the case. Some children will eat or drink anything that is at hand, fall from trees, ladders or bicycles, get bitten by every conceivable type of animal, push wires into electrical points, break their bones, get burnt or scalded, push objects in their ears or up their noses, swallow coins, toys and other objects. The list is endless.

Small children brought in as overdose patients created problems for the staff, as it was not always easy to do a stomach washout on a child. The casualty officer had to assess the possible effects of the substance that had been swallowed. Alcoholic beverages have a fascination for some children, and that special bottle father kept for himself on the top shelf of the cocktail cabinet might not be out of the reach of some inquisitive child.

William, who was twelve years old, and who came from

a middle class family, was found unconscious in his father's wine cellar clutching an empty port bottle. He was rushed to Casualty, and could well have died from choking on his own vomit if he had not been discovered. Fortunately he was found in time, and it was only when he was admitted to the Intensive Care Unit that his parents realised how ill he was. His father had previously treated the incident as a boyish escapade when he had described his son as having good taste, as it was a vintage port that he had downed!

The hidden dangers in the home take many forms. The storage of toxic solvents in bottles that have previously contained fruit juices or mineral water can be an invitation to the young to exercise their curiosity by tasting the liquid. Even if a child cannot read, if the original label is left on the bottle, the colours can tempt a child to drink some of the contents.

Parents cannot always be blamed for the accidents that their children are involved in. Some hard-working fathers and harassed mothers are trapped in their own environment, and it is virtually impossible to safeguard their children for 24 hours a day. All they can do is take all reasonable precautions.

* * *

Children always react very differently to hospital procedures, and before the renovation of the Accident and Emergency Department, there was no special section for young patients. They shared the same waiting room and treatment room as everyone else. It was the duty of the nursing staff to reassure the youngsters, but in spite of all the kind words and toys, the sight of the nurses' uniforms and the white coats of the doctors may have proved too overwhelming for some of them, and their screams and yells could be heard echoing through the department even before treatment had commenced.

Suturing young children could at times be difficult. Although some remained still and passive, others reacted violently and it was necessary to hold them down while the suturing was done. Very young patients were rolled in a blanket so that they could not move, but with older children it could take up to three of the staff to restrain them.

But kicking and struggling were not the only weapons in a child's armoury, as dear little Anthony could testify.

'Don't call him Tony, we insist that he be called Anthony,' his mother told Eve, the staff nurse who fetched him into the Treatment Room.

Dear little Anthony had a cut on his brow that merited a few stitches. But his mother was obviously concerned and she outlined to Eve all her son's past medical history, and described him as sensitive and frail. To me he looked bursting with health, with glowing cheeks and bright eyes and an air of youthful innocence. But if Anthony was a frail child, he was also a very spoilt one. He was crying and screaming all the time, which might have been understandable. But it was his demands for his mother's attention and her weak response that seemed to make the situation worse. That was the reason for my presence on the scene; I was there to help restrain him when Eve started stitching.

'Please don't hurt him,' said the mother. 'He's only a baby.'

'He's a big baby for a five-year-old,' said Eve. 'Don't worry, we won't hurt him. Just take a seat in the waiting room.'

'Can't I stay and hold his hand?'

Eve looked at me and gave a grin. Some parents were helpful and reassured their child while the suturing was being done; but others got very distressed, and there had been a few occasions when mothers had fainted in the Treatment Room, which had caused further problems.

'You'll be better in the waiting room,' Eve said, and ushered the mother through the door.

It is always distressing to have to suture children. Yet it is necessary not only for medical reasons, but also for aesthetic purposes, so no ugly scars mark the skin in later life. With Anthony it was not going to be an easy task. He was screaming, kicking and struggling as we laid him on the couch. I held his arms, but it was not enough, and Eve called a student nurse over to help us.

'Hold his legs and keep him still, otherwise I can't suture him,' she said.

Some nurses have a very good relationship with children, and Eve was included in that group. She seemed to gain their confidence with her calm reassurance, her friendly smile and her ability to put them at ease. But all her efforts with Anthony were in vain. He went on screaming and struggling, and every time we went near him he rolled his head from side to side, making it impossible for her to proceed.

'Keep your head still Anthony, please,' Eve pleaded with him.

Anthony replied with even more rolls of his head, and a greater volume of screams and yells. Both the student nurse and myself were having difficulties restraining him as he struggled and tossed his head from side to side. The energy that this "frail" boy generated, even at his early age, was quite amazing! We released our hold on him while Eve talked to him in her soft voice, trying to make him relax. After a few minutes we tried again, but it was to no avail; the struggles all started again.

It was then that the door opened and in walked Ken the porter. He stood and surveyed the room for a moment. His white coat with the red facings that denoted his status on the staff was unbuttoned as usual, and his sleeves were rolled up to his elbows, revealing the figure of a naked lady tattooed on the inside of his right arm, and part of a snake that disappeared up his left sleeve. He moved over to where Eve was standing, and said in a low voice that was nearly drowned by the patient's screams:

'What are you doing, trying to kill the poor little sod?'

The question went unheard by Anthony, but Ken's entrance was like an answer to Eve's prayers.

'Ken, you're just in time to give us a hand. Hold the patient's head for me while I stitch his brow, he just won't hold still.'

Ken looked rather dubious, but without a word he moved forward and by placing a hand on each side of Anthony's head, he stopped the movements immediately. The naked lady on his arm, who was showing her posterior, seemed to be taking an interest in the proceedings. Ken was very proud of that tattoo; by flexing the muscles of his right arm he could make her bottom move up and down. He called her Salome, and she was a great source of amusement to most of the children when he made her dance for them. Anthony, however, was not treated to Ken's little show, and I doubt that it would have made much difference in the present situation. All we wanted to do was get him sutured and send him home, as he was still screaming in his high-pitched voice.

'Are we all ready?' asked Eve as she stood gloved and waiting.

'Just a minute,' said Ken. 'I want to wipe my nose.'

It was a fatal mistake. He let go of Anthony's head, and the boy reared up and buried his teeth in the posterior of the tattooed lady on Ken's right arm. It was impossible to say who was the more surprised, the tattooed lady or Ken. The lady's eyes seem to widen with horror as she looked back over her shoulder, while Ken, who was never at a loss for words, seemed speechless for a while. He took a long deep breath and looked at Anthony, and in a voice loaded with menace he said:

'You little bastard.'

'Ken, please, you can't talk to my patient like that,' said Eve.

The student nurse gave a giggle, I sniggered and then we all dissolved into laughter. All, that is, except Ken, who stood examining his right arm, where Anthony's teeth marks were showing red on the bottom of the lady he loved. The boy had now stopped crying, and he was gazing with surprise as our laughter continued. It was Ken who took the initiative by grabbing the boy's head again, and in the same threatening voice he had used previously, he went on:

'Now lie still and shut your cake-hole, or I'll belt you one.'

It was doubtful if Anthony understood Ken's words, but I'm sure he recognised the implication behind them; apart from the odd whimper or two, he lay quietly and passive as Eve completed her suturing, and then finally gave him his anti-tetanus injection.

The last I saw of Anthony was when he was leaving in his mother's arms, going through the door asking her, 'Mummy, why am I a little bastard?'

I didn't wait to hear her reply. Perhaps he should have asked Ken.

* * *

Being somewhat naive in my approach to my fellow creatures, I always imagined little boys and girls to be simple children of nature, wide-eyed, rosy-cheeked and innocent, and endowed with love and affection. Most of them are, of course, but there are a few, just a few, who exist in our society who would try the patience of a saint, and who helped to destroy some of the illusions that I had about children. The workers in every casualty department are familiar with all the four-letter words that interlace the vocabulary of some of their patients. These emissions of bad language come mostly from the drunks and the ignorant who have no regard for the feelings of the people who have to listen to them. But there is another group too. Some of the most foul language I have ever heard came from the lips of small children. The tone of it I'm sure would have brought blushes to the cheeks of any N.C.O. in the British Army.

Although in most cases the child's upbringing must have been a contributing factor, it was not always the case. Some of the worst culprits came from upper and middle class homes, and had caring parents. One could only conclude in most cases that the four-letter words were in common usage by their families, and the children absorbed them.

One very small boy who was being treated by a staff nurse suddenly let out a stream of invective as she started to suture his cut finger.

'Do you call your mummy all those wicked names?' she asked.

'No,' said the lad. 'But daddy does.'

Man's humanity to man is always reflected in the patients that pass through the doors of any hospital, but one aspect of this, cruelty to children, is a blot on our society. In spite of the existing legislation and the increased awareness by our Social Services, it seems impossible to stop these incidents taking place. Some of these crimes may be committed through ignorance, and frustration, but there are some crimes which society should not tolerate, and this is when children are abused sexually. Battered Baby Syndrome is a term used by our popular press, but Shattered Mind Syndrome is never mentioned. This is equally revolting to members of the medical profession. Some children are so frightened and withdrawn when they are brought to hospital that it may take days before they speak to members of the staff. Through the cruelty they had endured, it was impossible to tell what mental scars would remain with them for the rest of their lives.

To combat cases of child cruelty, hospitals kept a register of suspect cases. These were filed under the heading of Non-Accidental Injuries, and suspect cases were cross-checked with the information on the list. The names of the patient's doctor, and social worker were also included so they could be contacted if necessary.

Hospital staff are not devoid of human emotions. They laugh when they are happy, and cry when they are sad, and the only difference between them and their patients is that they are supposed to hide their feelings and retain an outward calm at all times. But in one case it was different, and the whole of the staff were openly angry and appalled at the injuries and abuse inflicted on one small child.

Baby Mary was born to someone who did not want her. The child's mother, young and unmarried, put her into the care of one of her friends just after she was born and then, perhaps as a gesture against the male sex, became involved with a circle of lesbian companions. It may be that Mary found some stability in her early years, and perhaps affection, but when she reached the age of six, her foster father was sent to prison and his common-law wife entered into a new relationship with a man Mary called uncle. And then her troubles began.

The child was admitted late one Saturday night to the Accident and Emergency Department, accompanied by a policewoman and a social worker. She looked like a little elf as she lay on the bed, wide-eyed and innocent. In spite of her neglected appearance, she was a pretty child. She uttered no sound as she stared around the room, and her silence was not through shyness but fear. The staff tried to talk to her and reassure her. The medical examination continued for some time with a surgeon present, and then she was taken to a ward to be prepared for the operating theatre.

The facts about Mary slowly emerged. She had been abused from the front and rear by the man she called her uncle. Stitched and incapacitated, she lay in her cot, fearful of the nurses who were caring for her, and frightened by the laughter of other children on the ward. I saw Mary several times when I visited the ward, but she would not speak to me. Then one day she was gone. I never knew what happened to her, or of the fate of the man who had abused her, but I was saddened by the thought that there must be many children like her suffering from the same abuse, as people continue to turn their heads and look the other way when they hear a child's cry for help.

* * *

It was one of those cold Winter nights when the wind seemed to penetrate through the skin, and I sat with Len the night clerk warming my hands round a mug of tea. It was ten o'clock and it was the quiet period, too early for the usual Saturday night revellers and too late for most of the domestic accidents. It was a night to be at home by the fireside watching television, or curled up in a chair reading a book with a hot drink within reach.

The outside door of the Casualty Department was getting weary with use. It was perfectly alright during the warm weather, but in Winter the gap between the door and the frame was somewhat wider than we would have wished, resulting in a miniature hurricane blowing through the existing spaces in the woodwork. The spring on the door also refused to work through old age, so anyone entering the department during a very cold period was met with a loud cry of, 'Shut the door please, it's cold in here.'

This was the situation when little Fred made his first visit to Casualty. Len had turned his back to the counter to start filing some of the patients' cards when the door opened and a small figure walked in and the head of a young boy encased in a Balaclava helmet appeared just above the counter. Two bright eyes and a snub nose were visible through the holes in the helmet, and a hand was held upright with the fore-finger elevated pointing Heavenwards, like the gesture of the Pope when he blesses the crowds that gather in St. Peter's Square, or a cricket umpire hastening the departure of some unfortunate batsman.

I gave Len a nudge and he turned round from his labours. Leaning over the desk he managed to look down at Fred. In a serious sounding voice he asked, 'Can I help you, son?'

Fred looked at him. 'Are you a doctor man?' he asked.

'No. Did you want to see one?'

'Yes please'

'What for?'

'My poorly finger.'

Fred pushed his finger through the slot in the glass screen, and Len regarded it solemnly and at close range for a few seconds.

'What's the matter with it?' he asked.

'Can't you see?'

'Well, it could do with a good wash.'

'I've cut it,' said Fred.

There was another moment of slow scrutiny on Len's part and, still maintaining his serious look, he turned to me.

'I'd like a second opinion,' he said.

It was my turn to continue the examination, and I looked at the finger with great solemnity.

'I don't think it will be necessary to remove the finger, I'm sure a sticking plaster will do the trick.'

'Where's your mummy and daddy?' Len asked the boy.

'At the Club.'

'How old are you?'

'Nearly seven.'

'Well, you come back tomorrow and we'll put a plaster on your finger.'

'Don't be daft, I want to see the doctor man tonight.'

'I think I'd better find out who he is, and where he comes from,' Len whispered in my ear. 'He's too young to be wandering about on his own at this hour. Besides, it's bloody cold outside. Take over the desk, I'll have words with Sister.' He went into the corridor and, taking the boy by the hand, he led him towards the treatment cubicles.

It was some time later when Fred returned. This time he was escorted by Sister.

'Walter, would you mind running Fred home in your car? I can't use an ambulance and I don't want to get the police involved, but he's too young to walk back on his own at this hour. He lives in the council flats at the back of the hospital. His parents must be worried about him, but tell them we have given him some hot milk and biscuits.'

Fred had evidently not been in a car before, and he seemed quite thrilled when I allowed him to switch on the lights before I put the seat belt round him. When we reached the flats I followed him inside along a dimly-lit corridor until we reached a door that was splintered and scratched on the exterior as though someone had been kicking it.

'Is this where you live?' I asked. 'Do you have a key?'

As if to answer my question, he gave the door a good push, and it swung open. After knocking without any result, I followed him inside and called: 'Is there anyone there?' But there was no answer. The single electric light bulb that hung from the ceiling was still lit, and the smell of stale food, and animal odours, met my nose as I entered. A table covered with newspaper and piled with empty dishes stood in the centre of the room and a group of beer bottles, also empty, lay on their sides in a far corner. The room was bitterly cold, the gas fire was unlit, and the only source of heat came from a paraffin stove that stood smoking near the window. I was in a dilemma. I did not want to leave the boy alone, but I was an intruder in the flat, and if his parents were out at some club it might be hours before they returned. I looked at my watch. It was now half past eleven.

'Will you be alright now if I leave you, Fred?' I asked.

'Don't go mister, wait until my dad and mam comes home. I don't like being on my own.'

'Will they be long?'

'I don't know.'

'Alright, I'll stay for a little while.'

The little while was about thirty minutes. As I sat in a chair talking to Fred, the door was kicked open to herald the arrival of the missing parents. The mother entered first, the dim light highlighting her blonde hair with its dark streaks. She was wearing a very short skirt, and the long string of pearls twisted round her neck hung down to her waist. The fur coat that hung over her arm was ginger coloured; it reminded me of my neighbour's tom cat that always caused me so much trouble. She leaned against the wall for support as she came in. Her husband, or partner, who followed behind was a large man with a deep red face. I wasn't sure if his colour was caused by the cold outside or by his visit to the "club", wherever that was, but by the look of his burly frame he could have picked me up and thrown me through the window had he so desired. He stood blinking at me for a few seconds as I sat in the corner of the room, still wearing my white coat. The anticipated outburst was not long in coming.

'Who the bloody hell are you?'

'I've brought your son back from the Casualty Department at the hospital. He's had a plaster put on his finger, but it's not serious. I think he wanted someone to talk to. Sister did not want him out on the streets alone so she asked me to bring him home.'

'You little sod.' The man turned on the boy. 'I told you not to leave the flat. Get into your bed, I'll deal with you later.' A spate of four-letter words followed the boy as he scurried out of the room.

'Don't be too hard on the lad,' I said. 'He's a grand little chap.'

'Piss off and mind your own business. You bloody do-gooders are all the same.'

I stood for a moment and then, realising words were useless, I made my way to the door and turned to bid them goodnight. But the red-faced man was still uttering threats, while his wife had now collapsed in the chair that I had vacated, her ginger fur coat lying on the floor beside her.

Fred continued to make further late night visits to the Casualty Department. I did take him home on some occasions, but I dropped him outside the flats where he lived to avoid any intimidation from his father. Sister and the staff were aware that this was a case of child neglect on the part of the parents and so the social services were called in. I can only assume some action was taken, because Fred vanished from the scene, but we missed the red-nosed, bright-eyed little boy who had been denied the love that he should have received at home. Perhaps he found some affection when he came looking for his "doctor man".

* * *

'Are you a doctor?'

I stopped and turned to the woman who addressed me as I walked along the corridor leading to the consulting rooms and as I was wearing a white coat that I had purloined from the staff room, I suppose her mistake was understandable. The woman was shabbily dressed, and her hair was heavy with ironmongery that bulged out underneath the headscarf she was wearing. She was holding a small child in her arms that was wrapped in a tattered shawl. She wore a pair of yellow socks which clashed with the red slippers that encased her feet. They must have been too small for her as they had been slit at the top. I must have delayed answering, and she repeated the question. 'Well, are you a doctor?'

'No, why do you ask?'

'I want to see a doctor.'

'But you've just seen one. You were in his consulting room a short time ago.'

'I mean a real doctor.'

'He was a real doctor.'

'He was a bleeding witch doctor. He's a wog. I don't want him to examine my child.'

'Do you know what's wrong with her?'

'She's got measles.'

'How do you know?'

'I've had four kinds, and I should know when they've got bloody measles. She's been like it for three days now.'

It was now nine o'clock on a Saturday night. The night staff had just arrived to take over from the afternoon shift. I looked down at the small child in her arms. A tiny pink face protruded from the shawl, and the baby's arms were wrestling to free themselves from the wrappings, she was making whimpering sounds as she struggled.

'Shouldn't you have taken her to see your own doctor before now if you suspected that she had measles?'

'This is a hospital?'

'Well yes ...'

'Are you a nurse.'

'No.'

'Then you can't help me.'

'No, but ...'

'Then sod off and find me someone that can.'

I retreated towards Sister who stood at the end of the corridor talking to a staff nurse. This was a problem for her to solve.

You are likely to meet the most charming people in any Casualty Department, and being a voluntary worker I had to absorb all the abuse that was directed at me. I could not afford to get involved in areas that were covered by the professional staff. In a way I was often at the mercy of some of the most abusive individuals that I have ever met. Strong language and argument are poor weapons to use in return, as it only inflames a critical situation; but it is very difficult not to react in the same vein.

Another cardinal sin in the catalogue of cruelty to young children is the one of neglect. Physical injury can in some cases be inflicted on a child in the heat of the moment, but neglect is premeditated and intentional. It comes in many forms and cuts through every strata of our society, from poor parents who seek to drown their troubles in the local pub, or win a fortune in the Bingo Hall, to the golfing, bridge-club fraternity, who also leave their children alone, perhaps to enhance their status in society. Ignorance can be the cause of some forms of neglect, but selfishness is usually to blame. Parents put their personal pleasures before the welfare of their children, leaving them alone, often in filthy conditions, poorly clad and underfed. There are many degrees of neglect, and both the rich and poor are equally guilty of this crime.

Neglected children ranged from half-starved babies to lice-ridden youngsters who were brought into the hospital by the police or social workers during the course of the year. Their stories unfolded in the Casualty Department.

One young mother left her baby sleeping in a cot so she could go out drinking with her friends, and on her return she discovered that she could not wake the infant. When she got concerned about the child's breathing, she carried the baby to hospital for treatment, not realising that it was dead.

Paul was only a year old when he was left unattended in his cot for nearly two days. Unwashed and underfed, he lay in his own filth, and he probably owed his life to a milkman, who noticed that the previous day's milk delivery lay untouched. On hearing a child crying inside the house, he asked the police to investigate, and they made a forced entry, and Paul was brought into hospital, suffering from dehydration and lack of food. It was subsequently discovered that Paul's parents had quarrelled and walked out of the house, both of them labouring under the impression that their opposite number would look after the child.

I was an observer when such incidents occurred, and it was as though I was looking through a window at some strange unreal world passing before my eyes, a world remote from my own private existence. It appalled me that such cruelty could be inflicted on innocent children. It was not easy for the medical and nursing staff to remain neutral in their attitudes to cases of child neglect, for many of the staff had children of their own, and although they were there to mend the broken bodies or ease the minds of these young victims, and restore them back to health, they were outraged by the incidents.

Many cases of child violence, some resulting in the death of the victim, were reported in the press months afterwards, and when the accused were brought to trial, the dividing line between murder and manslaughter was often a point of law that was argued in court. The punishment never seemed to fit the crime, and it was strange yet somehow fitting that the real poetic justice was inflicted on the guilty inside the prison by the inmates.

The Welfare State tries to build a protective wall around the citizens of this country, and the very young and the very old merit special attention. But in spite of the vast sums of money being spent to improve our healthcare, and our standard of living, there will always be a section of our society who will slip through the net. It is a sad experience for the staff on a children's ward who know that their socially deprived patients that they have restored back to health are likely to be discharged and returned to the environment they came from, lacking in food, love and comfort: the three things that thy had briefly received in hospital.

* * *

The main radio link with the Ambulance Control that was located at the rear of the reception desk suddenly burst into a cacophony of static and human voices. There was a short pause, and then the penetrating voice of the controller at the other end broke through.

'Control to Casualty.'

Jo dropped her pen on the desk and reached behind for the microphone.

'Casualty, go ahead.'

'There's an RTA on the way with a young boy aged about six, he's suffering from multiple injuries. The ETA will be about ten minutes. Tell the staff to stand by.'

'Casualty to Control. Roger.'

Before the echo of the message had receded I turned

from the desk where I had been helping out to go and alert the staff, but there was no need. The Iron Maiden, who also happened to be on duty on this particular Sunday evening, was standing in the door listening, and before Jo or I could speak, she reached for the phone and started to inform the medical and nursing staff, and also the surgical unit, of the patient's impending arrival. She replaced the receiver and her eyes alighted on me.

'Put a Deans trolley into the ambulance bay, Mr Cockshaw.'

'Yes, Sister.'

As she did with the rest of the male staff, she always addressed me as Mr and never the informal Walter that was used by the other sisters and nurses. It was a command not to be ignored. The Deans type of trolley was unlike the standard ones that were in general use at that time, and we only had three. These were usually kept for serious injuries, as the patients could then be processed through various departments, particularly the X-ray unit, without being moved from the vehicle, thus avoiding any unnecessary lifting that could cause further distress.

The mood and tempo of a Casualty Department can change in a matter of seconds. A phone call, a collapse or a cardiac arrest can disperse the staff and change the pace of the department. After working there for a time it was possible to sense the tension. It was a strange feeling, an anticipation of the unknown, as the condition of the patient was not fully revealed to the staff until the ambulance doors swung open.

Dealing with the victims of road traffic accidents called for the greatest professional expertise from the medical and nursing staff, but I did assist them when I could by undressing some of the patients. But even this procedure required great care to avoid causing any unnecessary pain. Only with guidance from the staff was I allowed to help. I pushed the Deans trolley outside into the ambulance bay. One of the casualty doctors and the sister also hovered round the door, and Danny the on-duty shift leader of the porters, joined me. The estimated time of arrival of the ambulance had been wrong; it was not ten minutes but nearer twenty. I had time to change the blankets on several used trolleys before I heard the sound of a siren getting nearer. I pushed my way through the swing doors of the ambulance bay in time to see a police car with its blue light flashing cut through the intersection leading to the hospital, and guiding the ambulance that was close behind it. The high-pitched sound of the siren dropped to a wail and slowly faded away as it swung round and allowed the ambulance to reverse into the bay. The Iron Maiden stood with the doctor at the rear, as the driver opened the doors and assisted his colleague to lift the patient out on a portable stretcher. I pushed the Deans trolley forward and the young boy was then lifted on to the trolley by means of the canvas sheet he was lying on.

'Are either of his parents with him?' the Sister asked the ambulance man.

'Yes, they came in the police car.'

The trolley was rushed into the Resuscitation Room and a surgeon and two nurses joined the rest of the white-clad figures. I took my place at the foot of the trolley and started removing the patient's shoes, followed by his socks, that were red and sticky from the blood that had run down his legs.

'Don't move his feet. Cut his trousers off,' The Iron Maiden ordered.

I reached for my scissors and started to cut through the blood-stained cloth. The boy was wearing a pair of denim jeans, a material that resisted the efforts of my small pair of scissors, which were unsuitable for the task. As I struggled on I could feel the perspiration gathering on my brow and running down my back caused by the heat of the overhead lamps and my frantic efforts. It was almost as if the team were depending on me as I cut through the last seam of the patient's jeans and flopped them back for Sister to remove them. I caught a glimpse of shattered legs that looked like a mass of raw flesh and bone. I stood back from the trolley as I knew my limitations; my part in the procedure was now over and the young boy's life was in the hands of the doctors and surgeons.

The patient made little groaning noises, blood trickled from his ears and mouth, and his shallow breathing intermingled with an occasional gurgling sound as he struggled to survive. The surgeon was directing orders to the nursing staff as he worked and the duty anaesthetist and his assistant now joined the group at the head of the trolley. I picked up the remains of the boy's jeans that lay on the floor. Along with the rest of his clothing I put them in a plastic bag and placed it in a corner of the room out of the way. Working in Casualty, even at my level, one can sense the outcome of traumatic cases such as this. It was obvious that the young patient was going to die. I looked at the small pathetic figure, at his mangled body and realised that there was nothing much that anyone could do for him.

'Oh God, let him die quickly. Don't let him suffer.'

Prayers never came easily to my lips and when they did they were usually for someone else. The twilight of half believing in God yet invoking his name only in times of need somehow offended my conscience and left me with a sense of guilt, with a feeling that I was using Him for my own ends. But today it was different, I was silently praying for both of us.

'Dear God, let him die in peace.'

The medical and nursing staff were working at a frantic speed; blood specimen ... drip ... dressings ... oxygen. The team was in action fighting for a life, and I was praying for a death. It was not the first time I had prayed for someone to die. It had happened before during the war. It was in the desert with the sun bearing down from a clear blue sky. The shell fragment that had torn a hole in the chest of Gunner Smith and left him stretched out on the rocks and gravel in the wadi, where he had been sheltering at the time, could not have been a personal symbol of hate from the man who had directed the shell. War is a very impersonal game, and we were also engaged in the same exercise. Poor Smithy was just one of the losers. He lay at our feet, still conscious, the bloody area of his wound covered with flies. He turned his head and tried to speak, but only managed to make sucking sounds, causing the blood to flow out his mouth. One of his friends, not knowing quite what to do, lit a cigarette and tried to push it between his lips. It was a futile act, but one I understood; it was probably the only cigarette he had. It was a gesture of farewell, as we all knew that Smithy was going to die, and I prayed that it would not be long.

'Please God, let him go in peace.'

That was long ago, yet the memory of it had been recalled by a small boy on a trolley who was also going to die very soon.

The Iron Maiden looked up from where she was working and glanced in my direction.

'Mr Cockshaw, would you take the parents a tray of tea. They are in the side room. Tell them I will come and see them shortly.'

'Yes, Sister,' I replied, wondering if she would ever use my Christian name. She must have known it by now.

Making tea for distressed relatives was a task that I often performed. This allowed the nurses to continue on their more important tasks in the treatment rooms and cubicles. The offer of tea added a human touch to hospital procedures; but it was also a yardstick to measure the patient's condition, as tea was only served to the relatives of the seriously ill.

I never did understand the morality of the situation. It was as though I was administering the last rites to the living instead of the dying. Work, however, is always a useful form of therapy, and even the simple act of making a pot of tea can ease the tension that exists during such incidents.

I left the kitchen carrying the tray and walked along the corridor towards the small side room where the boy's parents were. The door leading to the waiting room was open as I passed, and there was an overflow of patients still waiting to be seen by the casualty officers who were engaged with the boy in the Resuscitation Room. I must have progressed a few yards when a sudden jerk on my white coat brought me to a halt. It was so violent that I nearly dropped the tray I was carrying, and I turned round to face an angry-looking man, separated from me by the width of the tea tray. He thrust his head forward and was so close that I could smell the beer on his breath as he spoke.

'How much longer have I got to wait?'

He was dressed in an old pair of flannel trousers that were badly stained at the front and corrugated with creases; a blue sports blazer that had seen better days hung down from his shoulders. Over-sized, it descended to his legs and gave the impression that his body was out of proportion to his limbs.

He repeated the question.

'Well, how much longer do I have to wait? I've been here nearly two hours and no one's bothered about me. I could bleed to death and you lot wouldn't care.'

He thrust his jaw nearer to me over the tea tray, and the dark stubble on his unshaven chin gave him an unwashed appearance. I stood for a few seconds regarding him. My thoughts were still concerned with a small boy on a Deans trolley, and in the circumstances, explanations and excuses were useless. I turned away without answering and his voice followed me along the corridor.

'...I don't know why I pay my bloody National Health money for you lot to sit on your arses and swill tea down you.'

The small side room where the boy's parents were sitting was also used by the medical staff during the day for meetings and consultations. It was furnished with a few chairs, a side table and a desk. Balancing the tray on one hand I knocked, turned the door knob, and pushed my way inside using my knee.

The late evening sun slanted through the window, trapping the minute particles of dust that floated in its rays, and highlighting the man and woman who sat in the corner of the room. I placed the tray on the side table and moved it over towards them.

'Sister has sent you some tea, she will be with you soon.' The boy's mother was sitting straight-backed in a corner chair, her eyes half closed, seeing nothing. Her face was grey and worn. As she sat, her arms entwined the shoulders of the man who was on his knees in front of her, his head resting on her breast, his smothered sobs breaking the silence of the room. Not knowing what to say, I poured the milk into the cups.

'Please help yourself to sugar.'

There was no answer. The woman's gaze did not shift, and her hands were now stroking the man's hair. I was trapped by my own helplessness. All I could contribute to this situation was a pot of tea, and an invitation for two broken-hearted people to help themselves to sugar. They also knew the further anguish that was to come.

As I returned along the corridor, Danny the porter was changing the blankets on the empty trolleys.

'How's the boy,' I asked.

He pursed his lips and shook his head as if there was no need for words. I turned to go away.

'How are the parents taking it?'

'They are very upset. The mother is holding up, but the father is heartbroken.'

'Well he's sure to be, isn't he? He's in the transport business, and the poor bastard backed his lorry over his own son who was playing behind it.'

He finished what he was doing and walked away, shaking his head. I stood transfixed, my mind and body numb, and for the first time I wondered if this was really the voluntary work I wanted to do. But it didn't last, a nurse's voice brought me back to reality.

'... Porter ... porter, please ...'

The nurse standing outside the Treatment Room saw me and beckoned.

'Oh, Walter, can you help me take this patient to Millers Ward if you're free?'

The work of the hospital had to continue. There was no room for emotion, only understanding, and it was fifteen minutes later when I returned to the Casualty Department with the empty trolley. As I stood changing the pillows, the door of the Resuscitation Room opened and the Iron Maiden and a group of people came out. The last to appear was a young student nurse, who looked pale and close to tears, and her distress could hardly have escaped Sister's notice. The Iron Maiden turned to her.

'Nurse, go and give a hand in the Treatment Room. There must be some patients waiting.'

She then marched off in the direction of the side room, accompanied by one of the doctors, where the boy's parents still kept their lonely vigil. I had witnessed this sequence of events before, but this time it had a special significance for me, and I did not envy them this sad mission.

'The bloody heartless bitch,' said a voice behind me. 'She has no feelings.'

I turned to find one of the porters, who was watching the back of the Iron Maiden as she disappeared along the corridor. 'She must have a heart of stone,' he went on. 'She's not human.'

Death in all its forms is a constant presence in any hospital, especially Casualty. It was the living bodies that now had to be cared for and treated, regardless of our personal feelings. There was work to be done to try and catch up on the backlog of patients who were waiting for X-rays and transportation to the wards, and for a time I was quite busy helping the porters. It was when I was passing the side room that I realised I had not removed the tray of tea that I had taken in for the boy's parents.

Without thinking, I pushed my way through the door and stepped inside. The dying rays of the sun had now transformed the room with a roseate hue that reddened the walls. The figure of the Iron Maiden stood silhouetted against the window; she half turned at my entrance.

'I didn't hear you knock,' she said, but her voice had lost some of its hardness.

'I'm sorry, Sister, I didn't know you were here. I've come to collect the tea tray.'

I moved forward to the small table. Two untouched cups of cold tea still remained where I had left them. I gathered them up with the rest of the pots and made my way to the door, half turning as I struggled to find the handle. It was then that I saw a tear glistening on the cheek of the Iron Maiden.

I let the door close gently behind me as I went out.

Chapter 11

The Old Ones

It's such a long long time from May to December
And the days grow shorter, when you reach September

The old lady was evidently in great pain. She lay on the trolley moaning softly when our hands reached the point of her injury, which appeared to be a fractured femur. Her thoughts were also occupied by other matters.

'I haven't changed my underclothes this week,' she said.

'Don't worry, dear, that makes two of us,' replied Tracey the staff nurse. 'Just lie still while we undress you.'

Undressing female patients was not usually part of my job, but on occasions I was requested to assist the nursing staff if the person was seriously ill or overweight, and lifting was involved. This particular patient must have been around fifteen stone, so my services were needed.

'What happened to you dear?' Tracey asked.

'I had a fall yesterday and I couldn't get up. I've been lying on the floor all night.'

The patient was cocooned in a mass of clothing, and this may have kept her warm through the chilly Spring night and prevented hypothermia. It was these garments that Tracey and I were struggling to remove. Coat, cardigan, jumper, dress and underskirt all came off and were dropped in a polythene bag lying at the side of the trolley. But there was more to come. A multiplicity of strange garments still remained.

'I should think we are about halfway there,' Tracey said. She was trying to unhook the patient's stockings from some large metal suspenders that were sticking out below a pair of pale green bloomers with elasticated bottoms, and which left ugly red marks on the patient's thighs. Meanwhile I continued to wrestle with the clothes on the top half, which was not easy, as we were trying to avoid causing the patient any further distress.

'You have a lot of clothes on. Have you been feeling cold?' Tracey said.

'Yes, I do get cold at night. I don't always get undressed, so I sleep with my clothes on.'

'Help me lift her bottom Walter, I want to get her armour off. Go gently.'

With the help of a student nurse who had now joined us, we succeeded in lifting the patient slightly. I had managed to remove most of her top garments, leaving her clad in a very dirty-looking woolly vest. Now, with our hands straining under the weight of her body, Tracey fumbled in the voluminous green tent of the old lady's bloomers, and just as my arms were about to give way, she gave a cry of triumph, and very slowly withdrew a pair of filthy looking corsets from inside them. The mixed smell of body odour and urine that accompanied the garment caused me to wrinkle my nose as the aroma enveloped the small cubicle before the corsets joined the other items in the polythene bag.

'I don't know what the latest fashions are in ladies' underwear,' I whispered in Tracey's ear. 'But I now know why it takes them so long to get dressed in the morning.'

'Don't be so bloody cheeky,' she whispered in return, and then turning to the patient she went on: 'We'll get the doctor to come and see you now. Do you have any relatives that we can get in touch with?'

'I'm a widow, but I do have a married son.'

'Can we send for him?'

'I don't know where he lives; he's moved to another

house, but he's a good lad, he brought me some flowers when he visited me at Christmas.'

Tracey looked across at me, and by the tilt of her head and the sharp intake of breath, I could sense her opinion of the "good lad" who had brought his mother flowers for Christmas, and neglected her ever since; we were now in the month of April. Most likely the old lady would turn out to be another unwanted parent, possibly dumped into the lap of the Social Services, another victim of our hit and run society.

Throughout the year our Accident and Emergency Department treated numerous elderly patients, many living in adverse conditions. Many of these were discharged unless their injuries or illnesses merited their admission to a ward, or if they were suffering from some terminal illness and had no one to look after them. These patients could at least live out the remainder of their days in a clean bed, and be allowed to die with dignity.

The hospital at that time had no geriatric unit, and so the elderly were allocated beds that were available in the general wards. But it could not offer any shelter for long-stay patients who lived alone and were rejected by their families. There were at times very strong reactions from some of the relatives when they were informed that a parent was going to be discharged into their care. In an ideal world, hospitals would offer all the care and attention possible for an indefinite period, but the hard facts of life are dictated by shortage of money, staff and beds. It brought no joy to the hospital staff to discharge an elderly patient, who usually lived alone, into the care of some bitter and insensitive relative. Very often the bonds of friendship extended beyond the hospital walls, and the nursing staff performed many acts of kindness for their elderly patients.

* * *

I had just arrived back from the X-ray Department when Fred the ambulance-man saw me. He waved his arm and beckoned me to the doors of the ambulance bay.

'Can you give us a lift?' he enquired as I approached.

'What's the matter?' I said. 'Are the members of the Ambulance Service all getting weak these days?'

'Weak be buggered. Wait until you see what we've brought in.'

I followed him into the ambulance bay and joined the group of people who were assembled outside. There were two ambulance-men, two nurses, two porters and the casualty officer.

'It looks as if you have got the whole of the Casualty Department here, Fred, you don't need me.'

'Just flex your muscles and stand by.'

Being curious, I followed one of the porters into the rear of the ambulance, and once inside I stared in disbelief when I saw Maggie for the first time. Well, you could hardly miss her, she was such a tremendous size. The lady lay on a portable stretcher, but only just; her body flowed over the sides in a sea of flesh, and her right side, which was pressed against the ambulance wall, rippled in waves when she moved. I was also overwhelmed on my entrance by the sickly smell of rotting humanity, a cloying stench of decay so overpowering it grabbed you by the throat and adhered to the skin. I stepped outside again and gulped some fresh air.

'Bloody hell,' said one of the porters. 'We need some barrier clothing before we lift her.'

'You'll need a gas mask as well,' said Fred.

Lifting Maggie out of the ambulance was a scientific challenge and it was a mystery to me how the ambulance-men had got her in; they must have had some help. The male members of the group, which included me, were now attired in theatre gowns, face masks, gloves and caps. The canvas sheet that

Maggie was lying on was not wide enough for her body, but with the aid of poles threaded through the sides of the sheet and a united lift, we staggered down the steps of the ambulance and managed to lift her on to a trolley. Her flesh rolled over the sides, making it impossible for us to lift the security bars to keep her in place. The smell seemed worse than ever, a mixture of sweat, urine and faeces, and my stomach revolted against the stench. I noticed one of the nurses looking rather shaken, and she shook her head in disbelief.

'She really does smell,' she said.

Fred, never a man to mince words, was more to the point.

'So would you if you had been lying in your own shit for weeks,' he said.

The truth of Fred's statement was realised later when under the direction of the casualty officer, two nurses, a porter and myself, we gave a hand to try and clean Maggie. The patient was in her sixties, and must have weighed about twenty stone. She was wearing some filthy underclothes when she arrived, and these had to be cut off her. Her body from the neck downwards was covered with open sores, and her torso was encased in her own dirt that must have accumulated over weeks. Her legs and ankles were so badly swollen that it was unlikely she had been able to walk. The ambulance crew who had brought her into hospital unfolded a story of appalling ignorance and neglect.

Maggie lived with a married daughter, occupying a spare room in her house, and she had been bed-ridden for an unknown period. No medical aid had been requested for her by her relatives, and she had been left in her own filth, unwashed, untreated bedsores and with no change of clothes or bed linen. If a neighbour had not intervened and called a doctor, it is unlikely that her condition would have been brought to light, and she could have died in circumstances that defy the imagination.

Using warm water and swabs to begin with, we washed the front of her body to remove the encrusted dirt, which revealed the tiny white mites that inhabited the open sores. The water in the plastic bowls that contained an antiseptic solution had to be constantly changed as we worked. Our barrier clothing did little to protect us from the smell that permeated through it. Trying to turn Maggie on her side so that we could clean the other parts of her body caused us further problems. We had no desire to cause her unnecessary pain, but with the aid of pillows and props, we did somehow manage to do it, revealing further the foul condition she was in. When the washing was done, the second process started as the doctor started treating her open sores.

Maggie never spoke at all, but whimpered at times when the hands that were treating her travelled over the worst affected parts of her body. She seemed to be in a semi-conscious state, and although the staff were talking to her she made no gestures or response, but remained in her own private hell. It all took quite some time, and after a final examination by the doctor, arrangements were made to admit her to a side room off one of the wards. Once again it was no easy task to move her, but with the aid of three porters and the lifting poles, we managed to complete the operation and get her into a special bed. I never saw Maggie again, and when I enquired about her the following week, the sister in charge of the ward gave a little shrug of her shoulders.

'She's beyond all pain now,' she said.

Perhaps Maggie had found the peace she wanted.

* * *

'Can you get a patient undressed for me, Walter?' the staff nurse asked as she came out of the cubicle, letting the curtain drop behind her. 'It's the man in there,' she gestured with her hand. 'His language is appalling, and he won't let me get near to him. He's got a leg injury, and we need to remove his trousers so the doctor can examine him.'

'I'll do my best, Staff.'

'You had better duck when you go in, he's inclined to throw things at you.'

I stepped inside the cubicle and the prone figure on the trolley suddenly came to life. Two hands grabbed the side rails, the patient heaved himself forward to an almost sitting position and looked straight at me. He evidently didn't like what he saw.

'If you come near me I'll wrap a bloody bedpan round your neck,' the voice said.

I halted and took two paces backwards. The voice came from a man in his late sixties, and although the front of his trousers was stained by mud, maybe the result of his accident, I could not help noticing his clean white shirt, closely shaven face and the neat parting in his receding hair. He still had on his pair of highly polished black boots that looked out of place with the brown jacket and trousers he wore.

'I don't have a bedpan,' I replied.

'You'll need one if you don't piss off and leave me alone.'

'We're only trying to help you. We want to get you undressed so the doctor can examine you.'

'I don't want you or the bloody doctors near me. I want to go home, so get me an ambulance.'

He was a big man, judging by his partly-sitting, partly-lying position, and he probably could commit mayhem with a bedpan, in spite of his age. His large hands clutched the side rails of the trolley, and the one nearest to me had a large blue anchor tattooed on a red background, with some indistinguishable lettering beneath it. I thought that I would appeal to his better nature – if he had one.

'What about the poor nurse outside?' She's got to take your blood pressure and do the observations for the doctor.'

'Tell her to get lost. I'm not letting any young wench look at my body. When my old woman was alive I wouldn't let her do what she wanted to do.'

He obviously didn't have a better nature.

'But she's a nurse...'

'Tell her to piss off.'

'You wouldn't have told her father to piss off.'

'What the hell are you on about?'

'Well, her father was a captain in the Navy. Weren't you in the Navy?'

There was a pause and his hands relaxed on the sides of the trolley. He lowered himself back into prone position.

'How did you know that I was in the Navy?' he asked in a much softer voice.

'By your tattoo. Besides, you can always tell an ex-naval man, they never lose their smartness. I bet you had a girl in every port?'

I stepped forward and started unlacing his boots. 'Which leg have you injured?'

'It's my left... Do you know anything about him?'

'Who?' I said, finally removing his footwear.

'The nurse's father. Do you know what ship he was on?'

I searched my memory for an answer to the question. I couldn't leave the subject now, I was getting on too well with the undressing procedure. I tried hard to think of the Navy ships that had berthed in the North African ports during my time with the Eighth Army, and I hoped I was not going to regret this fabrication.

'I did hear that he was on the Terror.'

By this time I had lowered one side of the trolley, and

was busy removing his outer clothing. I had managed to get his jacket off and was now struggling with his braces.

'The Terror, did you say?' He was now showing some interest.

'Er ... Yes. It had very big guns.'

'Of course, she had big guns, you silly sod. She was a Monitor. I knew her well.'

'Well that explains it now,' I said, hoping that this particular topic of conversation would finally cease. With a gentle tug I managed to remove his trousers, taking care to avoid causing him pain at the site of his injury. After folding his clothes and placing them beneath the trolley, I covered him with a blanket.

'Were you in the war?' he asked.

'I was with the Eighth Army.'

A chain of reminiscences followed. This common denominator acted as a catalyst and formed a bond between us. Battles were fought all over again, and the names of ships and men poured from his lips as he relived his past experiences. Just letting him talk seemed to have a great therapeutic effect on the patient. I wondered if he lived alone and, like a lot of elderly people, lacked the companionship of his former life.

'I shall have to go now,' I said. 'It's been nice talking to you. Let the nurse look after you, and don't swear at her, she's a very nice girl.'

'What's her father's name?'

'Her father?'

'The Captain.'

'Oh, the Captain ... er ... Jones,' I said, plucking a name from out of the air. There must have been thousands of Jones in the Navy during the war, and I raised my eyes to Heaven for forgiveness.

'Jones ... I wonder if it was that bastard Taffy Jones? He landed me in the brig on one occasion.'

'I don't know, you had better ask his daughter.'

A hasty retreat was now in order as the conversation was getting out of hand. I discovered the staff nurse standing near the store cupboard sorting through the dressings, and she looked up at my approach.

'Did you manage to get him undressed for me?'

'He's all yours, ready and waiting. You'll have no problems with him.'

'Thanks, Walter, I don't know how you managed it. He threatened me with violence if I went near him.' She turned towards the cubicles.

'By the way, was your father a captain in the Royal Navy?'

'A captain in the Navy ...? No.'

'And was his name Jones?'

'Of course not.'

'Well, it is now, if you want to stay alive when you go in there,' I said, pointing to the cubicle. 'You had better start dancing the Hornpipe.'

As I walked away, the nurse stared after me with a puzzled look on her face.

Well, she did ask me to get the patient undressed.

* * *

Mike, the Orthopaedic Consultant, came hurrying along the corridor carrying his brief case. He was a large man, and as his favourite sport was rugby, I could imagine him being very useful in the scrum. The little lady who was running at his heels and trying to keep pace with him was chattering away at high speed as he walked. I could not hear what she was saying, but Mike's head was nodding continuously as he strode along, as if in agreement with everything she was saying.

It was a quiet period in Casualty and the porters had

gone for a tea break during the interlude. I sat in a corner where I could view the activity going on around me. Mike, on seeing me, changed his pace and direction, came towards me and stopped to let the lady catch up with him. Her chattering stopped for a moment, then, taking a deep breath, she burst forth with another spate of words. Mike put his hand on her shoulder and, pointing to a vacant chair beside me, he turned to the woman.

'Sit down there dear, and tell this gentleman all your troubles. He's our resident counsellor and he will be very interested in your story. Start at the beginning.' He sat her down in the chair and winked at me.

'Thank you, Mike,' I said.

He gave a grin and made a quick retreat, leaving me with the woman. It was difficult to guess her age, owing to her drab appearance. She could have been in her sixties, but may have been younger, as her mode of dress and the dirt on her face and hands did not help in my assessment. Her clothes were stained and wrinkled as they hung on her, and the long black skirt she wore was coated with dried mud through trailing on the ground. The strong odour that surrounded her was a mixture of sweat and urine, and it assailed my nose by its close proximity. I though that I had become acclimatised to the smell of human bodies, sweaty feet in particular, but I was sickened by the smell.

'What's the matter, my dear?' I asked, trying not to get too near her.

'... as I was telling the doctor,' she went on, 'it's my neighbours.'

'Your neighbours?'

'Yes, they are trying to poison me.'

'What for?' A stupid question to ask.

'They want me dead.'

That's rather an extreme way to get rid of a smell, I thought.

'Why should they want to do that?'

'They are jealous of me.'

'Why?'

'It all started when the Queen came for tea.'

The little wheels in my brain started clicking into place, I had been elected as the departmental fall-guy for the night to entertain the time-wasters.

'Have you been to the police?' I asked.

'Yes, several times. I have a man guarding me.'

'What for?'

'The I.R.A. want to kill me.'

I thought it best not to question her too closely about this phase in her life, and I changed to listening instead of asking questions. As she went on chattering, I saw Tracey the staff nurse coming along the corridor towards me.

'Tracey!' I shouted. 'Can you help me?'

'Sorry,' she replied, and gave a broad grin. 'I'm busy. You are doing a grand job.' And she hurried off.

It was another hour before I finally managed to free myself of the woman by leading her outside, but not before I had learnt about the death of her canary, poisoned of course by the Russians; her visit to Buckingham Palace and her escape from Jack the Ripper. Parked alongside the wall was an old perambulator with a clutter of teddy bears inside, all sitting up, half covered by a dirty blanket. They all looked as soiled as their owner. She went over to them and murmuring endearments, she tucked the blanket round them and walked away.

'You were a great help to me in my hour of need,' I remarked to Tracey when I saw her.

She gave a laugh. 'Haven't you met poor Smelly Nelly before?' she asked.

'No, someone might have warned me.'

‘The poor dear is quite harmless, but we just haven’t the time to talk to her. It’s a sad reflection on our society.’

She walked away, leaving me to ponder on her words. How right she was.

Chapter 12

The Reception Desk

The telephone gave another long ring. I sighed and picked up the receiver.

'Accident and Emergency Department.'

There was a short pause, followed by a woman's voice.

'I want the Casualty Department.'

'This is the Casualty Department.'

'Then why do you call it the Accident and Emergency?'

I took a deep breath and left the question unanswered to avoid going into a detailed explanation. The simple reason was that the head of the department had issued instructions that the proper name for his domain should be the Accident and Emergency Department. However, the rest of the population were unaware of that fact, and to most people it remained the "Cas" or Casualty.

'The Accident and Emergency is the Casualty. Can I help you?'

'Have you had any accidents in today?'

'I haven't counted them but it must be well over a hundred.'

'Oh.'

'Can I help you?'

'I'm enquiring about our Fred.'

'Your Fred?'

'Yes. He went out about eight o'clock on his motorbike and he hasn't come home yet.'

I looked at the clock. It was now thirty minutes past midnight.

'Perhaps, madam, you could tell me ...'

'When I said he went out on his motorbike, it wasn't his really.'

'But I don't know ...'

'... it was his brother's. His own bike is in the garage, it needs repairing.'

'Could you please tell me...'

'It's going to cost him about fifty pounds. I told him to wait until it's been repaired but he wouldn't listen ...'

'Madam, will you tell me what his...'

'... so with him being so late I wondered if he had been involved in an accident, and I wanted to put my mind at rest, so I phoned you.'

'Madam, what's his name?'

'What did you say?'

'WHAT'S HIS NAME?'

'I told you his name. It's Fred.'

Working on the reception desk was an education. I was often used as a Missing Persons Bureau. Anxious relatives would phone at all hours to make sure that missing members of their families had not been mugged, murdered, raped or involved in a road accident. A quick check on the admission book usually provided a negative answer, and one could sense the relief of the person at the other end of the phone. Very occasionally, however, we did have admissions who were related to the person making the call, and in instances of this kind I always called a member of the staff to deal with the enquiry, as I was not allowed to pass on any information relating to patients, being a mere voluntary worker.

It was my usual practice to relieve the male night clerk on the reception desk so he could go for his break if there were no porters available, and even if there were, they usually passed the duty on to me. Dealing with drunks, anxious relatives and excited patients all clamouring for treatment, and trying to answer the phone at the same time was not a duty that appealed to the portering staff. The clerk on duty was open to abuse for every second some patients were kept waiting, and in the early days there was no protection against the more violent members of the public. It was easy to vault over the low counter, and assault the clerk, rip out the phones and cause other damage. A plate glass screen was fitted after one such incident, which gave a greater feeling of security, but at the same time it acted as a sound barrier, and must have given the impression that the hospital only employed deaf receptionists as we exchanged shouts over the counter. Fortunately this problem was overcome by making apertures in the glass screen.

With the arrival of each new patient, the clerk had to fill in a casualty card with details of the person's name, address, next of kin, type of injury or illness, their age, religion and the name of their G.P. These details were then entered into a master book along with the time of their arrival. It was always a tricky business to get this information from drunks, or patients that had overdosed on drugs, and some people would give false names and addresses for reasons known only to themselves. Certain members of the female sex were also reluctant to answer one particular question, as in the case of one lady.

'How old are you, Madam?'

Madam looked round at the other people waiting to be booked in and gave a simpering little laugh.

'Put me down as being over 21,' she replied.

I duly wrote down what she requested, but I inwardly assumed that 51 would be nearer her true age.

Working on the reception desk meant that you had to be prepared to face the unexpected day or night. During the early hours of one Sunday morning, I was sitting reading the previous day's paper. Alf the night clerk had gone for his usual break, and the department was relatively peaceful, that is until the

Man Mountain burst through the doors. He was a huge specimen of humanity, over six feet tall, with shoulders as wide as barn doors. His shirt was unbuttoned at the front revealing a chest matted with black hair, his sleeves were rolled up displaying the tattoos on his arms, and a leather belt decorated with metal studs and a big brass buckle kept his trousers secure. He was obviously an open-air type; even under the sickly lights of the waiting room his complexion had a brick-red appearance. In any situation he would have stood out as a menacing figure, and I sensed by his approach that he meant trouble. I was pleased that the partition divided us. Man Mountain looked down at me from the other side of the counter, and as he did so I noticed the set of his jaw, his clenched fists and a certain gleam in his eye. He looked somewhat upset, and this opinion was confirmed by his bellow that reverberated round the waiting room, and even woke old George, the tramp who was trying to sleep unobserved in the corner.

'Where is she then? Where is she then?'

This situation, I thought, called for a calm and cool approach.

'Who do you mean, Sir?' I put the stress on 'Sir'.

'Who the bloody hell do you think I mean. Where's my wife?'

'Your wife?'

'Don't sit there like a stuffed dummy, get off your arse and find her. I know she's with him.'

'With him ... with who?'

'Her fancy man. I'm going to kill the bastard. She told me she was spending the night at her mother's and I believed her.' 'What's your wife's name, Sir?'

'Brown. Mrs. Brown, Wentwell Street.'

'I'll check for you, Mr. Brown.'

I reached for the admission book and studied the list of

patients who had been admitted from early evening. No one by the name of Brown had recently been recorded.

'We don't have a patient by the name of Brown.'

'Don't bullshit me, she was in a car accident about an hour ago and one of my neighbours saw her getting into an ambulance.'

'Well I can assure you, Sir, that we haven't had a lady by that name admitted tonight.'

'Don't give me that load of shit, let me talk to the organ grinder, not his monkey. Who's in charge of this bloody place?' It was at this point that he started banging on the glass partition to emphasise his request, and I started praying that the hospital Works Department had made a good job of fixing it. Being a natural born coward, I beat a hasty retreat and found the person in charge, who happened to be Sister Sue.

Along with the other nursing sisters, Sue was always kind and compassionate to the patients under her care. Understanding as she was, however, she would not tolerate abuse or violence from anyone. She also had the reputation of being able to swear in several languages, and none of the four-letter words that were in common usage by some of the patients were strangers to her lips when the situation demanded. Five feet three inches high, her youthful appearance was very misleading – but she was no soft touch, and she could exchange abuse with any drunk and come out on top.

'What's wrong?' she asked as she joined me at the desk, and I explained what was happening. She re-checked the admission book that I handed her, and closed it with a snap.

'We don't have a Mrs Brown in here,' she said, leaning forward and speaking through the screen.

'Don't piss about with me,' replied Man Mountain. 'I know she's in here and I want to see her.'

Sue pulled herself up to her full five feet three inches,

unlatched the reception room door and entered the waiting area. Walking slowly up to the Man Mountain she looked up into his face and then, with an outstretched finger, she poked him in the region of his navel.

'Don't you bleeding well swear at me,' she said. 'I deplore bad language, and if there is any pissing about to be done, it will be on your part. You can piss off.'

I waited for the inevitable – one dead nursing sister, murdered in the course of duty.

'Now sit down,' Sue went on. 'Don't ever adopt such a violent attitude with me or my staff again. If you are worried about your wife, we will try and help you.'

To my amazement, Man Mountain sat down in a nearby chair. He had a shocked look on his face, and his mouth hung open in surprise. I don't think a woman had ever spoken to him before in such a manner. Sue confronted him at eye level as he sat.

'Where did your neighbour see the incident? I'll check with Ambulance Control.'

'Outside the city centre night club,' a meek voice answered.

Sue moved back behind the reception desk again and dialled a number on the phone. A whispered conversation ensued for a few minutes and after a while she put her hand over the mouthpiece and turned to me.

'Have we had any R.T.As. in during the last hour?'

'Yes, two patients suffering from shock.'

'What's their names?'

'Mr and Mrs Smith.'

'Well, they're going to get another shock now,' Sue said as she put down the receiver. 'Go and tell the staff nurse who is attending Mrs Smith to break the news to her that her other husband, Mr Brown, is here waiting to pick her up, and then tell Mr Smith that if he's got any bloody sense it's his turn to piss off.'

The messages were received as Sue had anticipated. Mrs Smith, or rather Mrs Brown, turned quite pale at the news, while Mr Smith suddenly had an uncontrollable urge to visit the toilet, and for some strange reason failed to return. Sometime later Sue escorted Man Mountain to the Treatment Room to be reunited with his wife, lecturing him as they went along the corridor. George the tramp relaxed again alongside the radiator in the corner of the waiting room, and went back to sleep as peace reigned once more.

Alf the reception clerk returned from his meal in the dining room. He sat down, stretched his arms and yawned.

'All quiet?' he asked.

'Yes, everything under control. Did you enjoy your supper?'

'The bloody fish was definitely off. I wouldn't even serve it to my wife's boyfriend.'

I'm sure Man Mountain would have other ideas.

* * *

The Grim Reaper is always at hand in every hospital, and never more so than in Accident and Emergency. He claims his victims swiftly. There is not always time for fond farewells, and all that is left behind is a legacy of pain and anguish for the family and friends.

Such was the case of a young motor cyclist who was brought in dead from a traffic accident one Saturday night at about ten o'clock. As there was no other vehicle involved; it was assumed that the driver, a young man in his twenties, had taken a bend too fast and collided with a tree. The tragic routine of identification of the body by his grief-stricken parents had been completed, and they had been driven home in a police car. It was now for the coroner to make the final judgement at the inquest.

The department was quiet, and Saturday night turned into Sunday morning. I sat alone at the reception desk in rather a sombre mood doing my relief duty. It had been a night of tragedy, with overdoses, cardiac arrests and traffic accidents, resulting in the porters making several visits to the Winter Gardens. I looked up as the door opened and two men walked in. In one way I was glad, as work would help to relieve my black gloom. They came to the counter, and I stood up from my chair to speak through the hole in the glass. I addressed the older of the two.

'Can I help you, Sir?'

He gestured towards the younger man by his side, who must have been in his early twenties.

'It's my son.'

'Is he ill?'

He looked cautiously at the young man, then turned again in my direction.

'He's very distressed, his friend was killed tonight in a motor cycling accident, a Mister Blank.'

I remained silent; the strict rule that prevented me passing on any information still applied.

'My son would like to see him.'

'Are you relatives, Sir?'

'No.'

'Then I'm sorry, I can't give you any information. I suggest that you get in touch with Mr. Blank's family.'

The son spoke for the first time. 'He was my best friend, we were at school together.' He pounded the glass panel that divided us with his fist, and shouted: 'I know he's in here. I want to see him.'

'Would you wait a minute, please?'

I moved over to the phone out of earshot and dialled the staff room for the Sister. I knew what the answer would be before I asked the question, but at least she would be aware of the situation that confronted me. It just wasn't possible to open the mortuary during the small hours of the morning, or at any other time, for people to view a body. The procedure of identification by relatives had taken place, which could be very distressing if the injuries on the deceased were visible. There was a strict code of ethics and the answer from Sister was a sympathetic but firm refusal.

'I'm sorry, Sir,' I went on, 'Sister is aware of your son's concern, but I'm afraid that it is not possible to see Mr. Blank.'

'He was my friend.' The panel shook again from the young man's fists. 'No one is going to stop me from seeing him.'

As the glass shook under his blows, the tears started streaming down his cheeks, and I was glad of the security provided by the screen. It was as if he was using it to vent his distress and frustration.

I addressed his father.

'Look, tell your son to sit down for a few minutes. I know he's had a shock, and I'll get him a cup of tea. If I was you, I would take him home.'

'He's terribly upset,' came the reply. 'He couldn't sleep, and then he started drinking, so I brought him here to try and pacify him. I'm sorry to trouble you.' He put his arm around his son's shoulders to comfort him.

'I'm going to see him... I'm going to see him,' the younger man raved and thrusting aside his father's arm, he ran to the door and pushed his way through.

'Go after him, Sir, and see if you can calm him down. He's in a bad emotional state, bring him back and let him sit down, I'll get a nurse to talk to him.'

The father walked over to the door. 'He's not usually like this, it must be the shock.' He shook his head and went outside.

As he disappeared, peace reigned once again. The phones were still silent. It had been a strange night so far, somewhat quiet. There had been no enquiries for any missing husbands, frivolous wives or wayward sons or daughters, and I wondered how long it would last.

I found out about ten minutes later. Ernie the porter burst through the doors panting; he had obviously been running, which was rather strange, as Ernie never ran. He could hurry at a fast walking pace at times when there was an urgent need, but to run was against his religion. He was a portly figure, and he regarded people who indulged in any form of physical exercise as material for an early grave. But he had definitely been running, and he leaned on the counter sucking air and trying to speak. It must be urgent, I thought, as he stood panting. Then the words came out.

'For God's sake, phone the police. I've just been over to the Maternity Wing and some daft bastard is trying to break into the mortuary. He's trying to kick the door open. I'll get Sister.' He dashed away to find her – well perhaps he didn't dash, it was more of a trot.

Looking back, it must have been a unique incident in the annals of the local police force. I could imagine the situation in their Control Room as the night's events wound down. The staff would have been relaxing over their cups of tea when they received my phone call on the direct line we had to their Control Room. The conversation that ensued will forever be engraved on my memory.

'Control Room, P.C. Brown.'

'This is the Accident and Emergency Department. Can

you send someone round urgently, there's a man trying to break into our mortuary.'

There was a long pause.

'Did you say trying to break into your mortuary?'

'Yes.'

'You don't mean trying to break out, do you? Ha! Ha!'

'For God's sake, send someone.'

I could hear bellows of laughter from the other end.

'What's your name, Sir?'

'Cockshaw – Walter Cockshaw.'

'Hold on, Sir.'

There was another pause, and I grew even more impatient. Then the other phone on the desk started ringing. At first I ignored it, but the ring seemed to grow in intensity, so I laid down the receiver and picked up the other one.

'Accident and Emergency.'

'Sergeant Green here, Police Control Room. We have some bloody idiot on our line who says there is someone trying to break into your mortuary. I thought I'd better check.'

'Yes we have, Sergeant, and I'm the bloody idiot. Get some of your people over here, all hell's breaking loose.'

There was a click at the other end, and I replaced both of the receivers. As I waited, a stream of porters and staff made their way through the door in the direction of the mortuary. To say that a state of panic existed would be wrong. Hospital staff are trained not to panic, but on this occasion they got very close to it. The Senior Nursing Officer followed by the Sister were the next to exit as I stood and watched from behind the desk.

Ron the night clerk came slowly through the door after his break, with the previous day's newspaper tucked under his arm. He gazed round the empty waiting room.

'It's all very quiet tonight.'

'It certainly is, Ron.'

As if on cue, two police cars pulled up outside the building with their blue flashing lights reflecting through the windows. There was the sound of slamming doors and excited voices.

'I wonder what's going on out there?' Ron asked.

'There's a man trying to break into the mortuary.'

'Oh yes.' He turned and put his newspaper in his locker. Then he stopped suddenly.

'What did you say?'

'There's a man trying to break into the mortuary.'

'Pull the other one. One of these days someone will believe you.'

As if to convince him, the doors opened and a host of people swarmed in, led by three policemen who were escorting the young man who had so dearly wanted to see his dead friend. He had to be the prime suspect in the incident. The boy's father, along with Sister and the nursing officer, followed on behind in heated conversation, trailed by the porters and even some of the domestic staff. Ron regarded them in amazement.

'Bloody hell!' was all he could manage.

There is always a very thin line between laughter and tears in our lives, and this scene could be played as a tragedy or comedy. The enquiries continued until the early hours of the morning, with the addition of the hospital Chief Administrator who had been called from his bed to join the enquiry. It was later revealed that the young man had obtained access to the mortuary, but had then been restrained by the porters, and apart from a splintered door no further damage had been done. The fact that the man knew where the mortuary was puzzled the staff, as it was not easily located by outsiders. It was assumed he had been employed by a contractor who had done work for the hospital, and he knew the layout of the area.

I never discovered what happened to the man concerned,

and on my next weekly visit to the hospital the incident was not mentioned. Perhaps it was better forgotten for the sake of all concerned.

* * *

In the late evening and the early hours of the morning, it was not easy for the more sensitive female patients to give the reason for their visit to a male receptionist, or to describe the more intimate details of their bodily functions. But we needed to complete the appropriate section in the casualty card, which was headed "Nature of illness or injury". When I was alone on the desk, I could understand their reluctance, although I had long reached the stage of accepting the unacceptable, knowing that the feelings and the confidentiality of the patients must always be respected.

One Saturday night, while I was busy filing away the finished casualty cards, I noticed two girls standing near the wall and whispering together, occasionally glancing in my direction. When I had completed the task a few minutes later, they were still there, and instinctively I asked the inevitable question.

'Can I help you?'

The two girls looked at each other and slowly advanced to the counter. There was another whispered consultation. The taller of the two leaned forward on the counter and in a hesitant voice said: 'Can my friend speak to a nurse, please?'

'Certainly. I'll fetch one for you.'

She did not specify whether it was a male or female nurse she wanted to speak to, as we had both on duty, but from experience and common sense I knew it would be the latter. By chance it was Sister Sue herself who ultimately came to the desk to see the girl and I moved as far away as possible and pretended to be busy so as to cause the patient no embarrassment.

'Now, what's your problem?' Sue began.

A one-sided conversation went on through the screen as the girl whispered the answers to Sue's questions. It was then that Sister's voice broke out loud and clear.

'How long did you say?'

The reply was whispered again.

'Six weeks?' said Sue. 'Are you seriously telling me it's been six weeks?'

The smaller of the girls was now in tears and she could only nod her head.

'Have you been to your own G.P.?'

Another nod and another whisper.

'Alright, dear, we'll get the doctor to see you. No wonder you're in pain. Book the young lady in, Walter, and bring her along to the cubicles.'

'What complaint do I put on her casualty card, Sister?' I asked.

'Constipation,' she replied as she walked away.

Two hours later I was sitting in the Staff Room drinking a well deserved cup of tea before going home when Sue walked in.

'What happened to the young girl suffering from constipation?' I asked.

'Oh, the doctor had her X-rayed.'

'Have you had the results yet?'

'Yes, she's got shit coming out of her earholes.'

The young student nurse who was sitting next to me looked shocked, but her interest was aroused.

'What treatment would you prescribe for that, Sister?'

'I'd put a stick of dynamite up her arse, and stand clear,' said Sue.

If some people were ultra sensitive about their complaints, other patients were not so fussy.

'What's your problem, Sir?' This was to a man whose unshaven face looked at me from the other side of the counter. He grinned, exposing blackened teeth, and his bad breath assailed my nostrils in spite of the intervening screen.

'I want to see a doctor.'

'Yes, Sir. What exactly is troubling you?' I asked, reaching for my pen.

'I've got a dose.'

'A dose?'

'Yeah ... A dose of syph ... the pox ... V.D.'

The people in the queue behind him all took a pace backward.

'I'm sorry, Sir, you will have to attend our special clinic on Monday. You can't get any treatment here tonight. I'll give you the details.'

'I want to see a doctor now.'

'I'll get a member of the staff to come and have a word with you. This is an Accident and Emergency Department.'

'Well, my dose was an accident.'

'It may well have been an accident, but it's not an emergency.'

The fear of venereal disease brought patients to us at all hours, but there was little the staff could do for them apart from directing them to the clinic that specialised in sexually transmitted diseases. The social implications of this type of disease had quite an effect on some of the people who suffered from them, causing them deep embarrassment and depression. In their minds it was as if the whole of society was passing moral judgement on them, while the department was in fact only acting as a clearing house for information.

Very often the patient would telephone, pretending to be

calling on someone else's behalf. They would ask such questions as 'I wonder if you could help my friend, he thinks he has V.D.'. It was always 'the friend' that was suffering from the complaint and never the caller, and many people enquiring were under the impression that they could be treated in the Casualty Department at any hour of the day. In spite of all the government's health education, it was surprising at that period how ignorant the general public were about venereal diseases. The receptionist in any casualty department is never quite sure what to expect when the telephone rings.

'Accident and Emergency Department. Can I help you?'

'I hope so, old man.'

'What's the problem, Sir?'

'We're in a bit of a fix.'

'Can you enlighten me please?'

'It's a somewhat delicate matter.'

'The staff are quite used to dealing with delicate matters.'

'Well, we have been conducting sexual experiments ... and er, well ... you know.'

'Know what, Sir?'

'One of the ladies has got an object stuck in her bodily aperture.'

'Can she walk, Sir?'

'With some difficulty.'

'I'll get one of the staff to talk to her.'

'Oh no, I want your advice.'

'I'm not qualified to give advice. I suggest you call an ambulance.'

'Will you send one along for her?'

'I'm sorry, I can't do that. You will have to ring for one. Dial 999.'

But the caller hung up, and although I alerted the Sister in charge, the patient failed to appear. Perhaps the offending object had somehow been removed, otherwise the person concerned would have encountered some difficulties when she had to use the toilet.

Enquiries by phone covered a whole range of subjects: dog bites, toothache, falls, overdoses and illnesses were among the more common problems. But there were many more queries from worried people. Some asked if we could supply the Morning After Pill, and with the advent of AIDS, many anonymous enquirers rang up seeking advice. Although I knew the answers to most of the questions people asked, I always passed them on to the qualified staff.

One night, when Sister Sue was on duty, I went to consult her on behalf of an anxious mother who had phoned for advice. I found her in her office with her feet resting on a chair opposite her, and her flat-heeled shoes on the floor at different angles, as though they had been kicked off. She looked up as I entered. 'My bloody feet are killing me,' she said, and after a pause: 'What the hell do you want now?'

'There's a lady on the phone, Sister, and she says that her young daughter, aged six, has swallowed all her birth control pills. She wants to know what to do.'

'She's started early.'

'What shall I tell her?'

'Tell her to give the child copious draughts of cold water, and sleep in the spare room tonight.'

I thought it more tactful to leave out the last piece of advice.

* * *

There is no great division between tears and laughter, and when a situation merits it, the hospital staff can smile or sympathise accordingly. The important factor is to laugh with people, and never at them.

I was sitting alone at the reception desk one Saturday night, reading one of the old magazines that members of the public were apt to bring to the hospital by the carload. In spite of their kindness, I was sure some of the donors must have been labouring under the impression that the patients, while confined to their beds, were anxious to catch up on events and stories that were five years old. Some of these contributions came from people who were moving house, or had been clearing out an attic and thought it a pity to throw the magazines away.

When the door opened I looked up and saw a well-dressed young man make his way to the counter. He wore a blue suit with a matching shirt and tie, his dark hair was neatly parted and I guessed he was in his late twenties. His appearance commanded respect, and I stood up from my chair and went over to the desk.

'Hello, Sir, can I help you?'

There was a short pause, and he wrinkled his nose as if to register disgust. Then in a cultured voice he said, 'Can I see a doctor?'

'What exactly is the trouble?' I asked as I reached for a casualty card to book him in.

'I've swallowed a tombstone.'

I looked at him. He seemed quite normal, and with his mode of dress and tone of voice, he seemed to be of a much better background than some of our usual patients who came in after the midnight hour.

'What have you swallowed, Sir?'

'A tombstone.'

One of the fundamental principles of medicine, so I am told, is to reassure the patient, but this was a new experience for me. Did I have to reassure him that he had not swallowed the tombstone, or that he had? Ask a silly question and expect a silly answer.

'Was it a large tombstone, Sir?'

'It was a reasonable sized one. I had some difficulty getting it down.'

'You had better sit down, you must be feeling ill.' I indicated the chair on the other side of the counter. 'I'll have a word with the Sister in charge. What's your name, Sir?'

'Steven Soggins.'

There were two Sisters on duty that night, and I managed to catch Jan, who happened to be in the Treatment Room checking the contents of a cupboard. Jan was a jovial type, and always helpful if I had any problems while I was in charge of the desk at break-time. But she had a persuasive manner when dealing with awkward patients, which her cheerful ways and ready smile belied.

'Can you come to the desk, Sister?' I asked.

'What's wrong, Walter?'

'I've got a real nutter who wants to see a doctor. He says he's swallowed a tombstone.'

'Jan gave a sigh. Closing the cupboard door, she turned to me.

'Do you know his name?'

'Steven Soggins.'

'Oh my God, not him again. The last time he came in he said he had swallowed a bus. He had as well. It was a small one from a Christmas cracker. Get his previous records out – you'll find them in the files – and book him in.'

Steven Soggins was certainly listed in the files. Over the previous six months he had swallowed coins, metal washers, bottle tops, plastic objects (unspecified) and even a spoon, also presumably out of a Christmas cracker. But there was no mention of tombstones. If ever there was a candidate for the Guinness Book of Records, then it would be Steven. I made out another casualty card and wrote: "Swallowed foreign body" in the appropriate column, then escorted him to the cubicles where Jan was waiting.

When I saw Steven again he was on a trolley at the end of the corridor near the treatment area, waiting for the results of his X-rays. At the other end was the porter's station, and the shift leader was Jack. A huge man at least six feet three inches tall, broad-chested and muscular, he seemed to tower over his staff. He stood talking with his hands in his pockets and his feet apart, which was his usual stance.

As I stood changing the blankets on the trolleys, I could sense a spirit of rebellion among the portering staff. Some of the men were arguing with the shift leader about who should do a certain job, and tempers were getting frayed. Jack was rapidly losing his patience and finally, turning to the porter on his left, he burst out: 'Don't bloody well argue with me, get on with the job.' And he turned his back as if to conclude the matter.

The porter, smarting from a sense of injustice, stormed along the corridor in the direction of Steven Soggins, and it was then that things started to happen. Seeing the porter approaching, Steven climbed down from his trolley and stood for a second or two clad only in his multi-coloured briefs. Then, swinging a blanket round him and holding it with his left hand he raised his right hand in salute as he stood in the path of the oncoming porter, and stopped him in his tracks.

'What the hell's the matter with you?' the porter began.

Steven, with his head held high and his arm outstretched in salute, addressed him in regal tones.

'I am from the Starship Enterprise. Take me to your leader.'

The porter didn't hesitate. 'That's the silly bugger down there,' he said, pointing to Jack at the other end of the corridor. 'Go and talk to him.' And he pushed his way past Steven, still muttering under his breath.

Giving the blanket another twirl, Steven glided along the corridor, his head still held high like some emperor from ancient Rome on a royal walkabout. I stood fascinated by the scene; it was going to be a very interesting confrontation and I could almost predict the outcome.

Jack still stood with his hands in his pockets and with his back to Steven. He was unaware of the figure behind him, and gave a jump when a loud voice bellowed in his ear.

'Hail to you!'

Startled, Jack swung round to face Steven, who was still wearing his blanket like a toga.

'I am from the Starship Enterprise, I salute you.'

Jack looked down on him from above; he was in no mood for playing games.

'F..k off you silly sod,' he said, and turned his back on Steven and walked away.

Steven wilted on the spot. He slunk back along the whole length of the corridor, trailing his blanket behind him, then climbed back on his trolley and faced the wall. He refused to speak to anyone else for the rest of the night.

I never did find out if he had swallowed a tombstone.

* * *

'Can you help me?'

The young man in a pair of green overalls moved nearer to the glass screen to make himself heard.

'I'll do my best,' I replied.

'I'm here on an emergency call to service a refrigeration unit that's not working properly, and I don't know where it is, or who to report to. The usual service engineer who looks after the hospital is on holiday, and I'm covering for him. Perhaps you could find out for me where I'm needed?'

Sunday night was always a difficult time to get any maintenance done, and most repair work was left until Monday, so I guessed this particular job must be urgent.

'If you would like to take a seat, I'll see what I can do for you,' I answered.

Reaching for the phone, I dialled the Porters' Lodge, and a voice I recognised as Danny's, the shift leader, answered.

'Are you expecting a service engineer, Danny, to work on a refrigerator? I've got a man waiting at the reception desk who says he has been called in to do some repair work.'

'Ah,' came the reply, 'I'll come and collect him. It's a breakdown in the Winter Gardens. I'll be there in about five minutes.'

Replacing the receiver, I turned to the engineer.

'You are expected, someone will be down to show you where to go. I gather that one of our units is not working properly?'

'Is it a cold storage one?'

'You could say that.'

'What do you use it for, meat storage?'

'You could say that.'

'If it's frozen it should be alright to eat, it'll keep.'

'I don't think so,' I said.

'You can take my word for it, I do a lot of work for butchers and people in the meat trade.'

'We have a lot of them here, but we have a different name for them.'

'Meat dressers, I suppose, like the people employed in the supermarkets.'

'A few of them too.'

The conversation was getting more ridiculous by the minute, and by the time Danny appeared on the scene, rattling a huge bunch of keys, the service engineer was expounding the basic theories of refrigeration and explaining the relationship of temperature control and the expansion of gases. I interrupted him to introduce him to his escort.

'We've been waiting for you,' Danny said.

'Well, I'd better get on with the job or I'll be here all night.'

'Right. I'll take you down to the mortuary.'

'The where?'

There was panic in the young man's voice, and the colour drained from his face.

'The mortuary.'

'Do you mean to say that I've got to work in the mortuary?'

'That's where you're needed.'

'Alone?'

'Well, you won't really be alone, there are plenty of people down there.' Danny gave me a sly wink.

'Dead people?'

'Well, they're not exactly singing and dancing.'

'I'm not doing it ... I'm not working with dead people.'

'Don't worry, you won't be getting any help from them.'

'You'll have to get someone else. I'm not doing the job.'

'Come and have a cup of tea and let's talk things over. I can guarantee you won't see one dead person while you're down there, they will all be out of sight, and one of my porters will be with you. My lads like the peaceful atmosphere of that place.' Danny took the engineer's arm and led him to the Porters' Lodge, and the young man's protests followed him as he walked away.

'I'm not doing it... I'm not doing it ...'

It was two hours later when I saw Danny again.

'Did he do the job?' I asked.

'It was the fastest bit of work I've ever seen,' he replied.

Chapter 13

Stop the World, I Want to Get Off

Sunset and evening star;
And one clear call for me!
And may there be no moaning of the bar,
When I put out to sea.

The soft strains of the orchestra filtered through the wide doorway and intermingled with the hum of guests' voices as they waited to be greeted by the two distinguished dignitaries who were waiting to receive them. As I joined the group I took some deep breaths and filled my lungs to relieve the tightness of the trousers round my waist, but the pull of my dinner jacket increased and I came to the rapid conclusion that I had really put on weight. It was time for me to start slimming and take more exercise, or alternatively buy a new evening suit.

Charity Balls were not really my scene, but I could not resist the invitation that had been extended to me by my charming companion, especially when it was accompanied by such a lovely smile. We slowly moved forward and after being announced, we shook hands with Mr President, resplendent in his chain of office, and moved on again to be introduced to his wife. As I extended my hand to her, I saw the small furrow of her brow and the slight wrinkles round her eyes as she studied my face.

'Good evening, Mr. Cockshaw,' she said, and looking directly at me she went on: 'Haven't we met before?'

'I think not, Ma'am,' I said, 'otherwise I should have remembered the occasion.'

I was trying to play the gallant gentleman and I don't know if I succeeded, but she smiled and I moved on.

But it was a lie. I had met her before.

Tonight she was dressed in a beautiful white gown that contrasted with her gleaming black hair. She wore some simple jewellery that really flattered her, and as she stood under the chandelier, her delicate skin was highlighted by just a touch of discreet make-up that enhanced her beauty. She stood tall and confident as she greeted all her guests with a charming smile. As I moved forward with the other guests, my thoughts returned to the last time we had met. It was in the Gastric Lavage Room in the Accident and Emergency Department, and I was helping the staff nurse to do a stomach washout. On that occasion the lady concerned was not arrayed in a lovely white dress but in a paper gown, and she was lying on her side on a trolley. Both her arms were behind her back, and I was holding them to restrain her so that she could not pull at the tube that was down her throat. Her dark hair was spread over the paper sheet and she was making choking noises as the staff nurse tried to reassure her.

'Try and relax. Take some deep breaths, and don't bite on the tube.'

Vomit was trickling from the corner of her mouth, and a student nurse who was standing at the head of the trolley was busy with a suction tube, trying to remove it. As the staff nurse worked away at flushing out the stomach, parts of the undisolved tablets were visible through the transparent plastic tube, along with the undigested food that she had eaten previously. The smell of alcohol was also apparent, and the contents were drained into a bucket on the floor by the side of the trolley. The patient had obviously been drinking either before or at the time she took the overdose, and this was not unusual in this type of incident. Many would-be suicides fortified themselves with alcohol to help pluck up enough courage to take the final step.

This patient was lucky, however, and although she had been serious in her intentions to kill herself, fate took a hand, and she was given the chance to live. The unexpected return home of a member of her family, and the discovery of a suicide note just after she had taken a full bottle of tablets, started a sequence of events that reached a climax in the Accident and Emergency Department. The reasons why she did it were not the concern of the staff; that could be determined later by other people. They were there to save her life, not to hold an enquiry.

But tonight she was truly alive, and she added charm to the gathering as she moved around among the guests, chatting and smiling. No, dear lady, perhaps I was wrong. It must have been another you I had met before.

Gastric lavage or the stomach pump, as it was commonly known, was used where possible to wash out the toxic contents of the patient's stomach. There were times when this procedure could not be followed, for example on unconscious patients and very small children who had accidentally swallowed dangerous liquids or substances. They were difficult to treat. I always regarded stomach wash-outs as an assault on the person concerned, as in most cases the patients had to be restrained from the normal reaction of struggling to take out the plastic tube when it was put down their throat. But it was a necessary procedure that was prescribed by the doctor, though usually carried out by a staff nurse, unless there were complications in the patient's condition.

Although gastric lavage procedures varied from time to time, the patients were usually turned on to their sides, generally the left, and the top of the trolley was tilted so the patient's head was at a lower level. Any dentures were removed, their arms were placed behind their backs and held by a porter to avoid the initial reaction when the tube was inserted in the mouth. Pinning down the patient was not always necessary, as some patients were quite passive. A few of our regular overdoses would even take the tube and swallow it without any guidance or advice from the nurse in charge. For most patients, however, the worst moment was when they were asked to swallow the plastic tube, as it generally resulted in vomiting, and it was then a suction tube was used to remove the vomit from their mouths. Very often patients were sick down the legs of nurses who were treating them, and this did not endear them to the staff. But it did add to the nurse's awareness when dealing with overdoses, and they made sure they were wearing long plastic aprons and overshoes when they had a repeat performance.

A sample of the patient's blood was sent to the Pathology Department, and some of the contents from the stomach were retained. Before the serious business of the washout began, jugs of tepid water were at hand for the staff nurse, and a funnel or a large plastic syringe was fitted to the end of a clear plastic tube. After the tube had been swallowed by the patient, the water was then gravity fed through the funnel by holding it high, or forced through by the syringe into the stomach. When the water had been absorbed, the funnel or syringe was then removed and the tube lowered. This allowed the water to flow back into a bucket on the floor, and bring out the toxic substances. This procedure was then repeated until the staff nurse was satisfied that only clear water was returning through the tube. Very often the washout took longer than anticipated, owing to pieces of undigested food blocking the tube, and these obstructions had to be cleared.

The management of patients suffering from drug overdoses was usually done by the casualty officer working to procedures that changed from time to time. Gastric lavage was recommended "for all conscious and semi-conscious patients who are thought to have taken an overdose, after making sure that their airway is clear".

For patients who had overdosed on tricyclics or aspirin, it was recommended that they should be washed out within six hours, and salicylate levels should be checked for four and six hours afterwards; while for a high ingestion of paracetamol and other drugs, it should be done within one hour ideally. But it was necessary to deal with each case individually, and consultation with the registrar was advised if any uncertainty arose. Other patients could be given activated charcoal orally if they had taken a potentially harmful drug; it was considered that the use of emetics, such as ipecac syrup to make the patient sick, should be discarded, apart from their limited use for overdoses in children. Charcoal was more appropriate as it prevented reabsorption.

There seemed to be no limit to the range of commodities and solvents that people would swallow, either by accident or deliberately, and it was not uncommon for some patients to be treated for overdosing several times in one week. These people were usually suffering from some mental disorders, and well known to the staff. They were usually greeted with dismay, as they required urgent attention, and doctors and nurses had to be diverted from attending to other patients to treat them.

Apart from tablets, domestic liquids found in most homes were at hand for some patients to consume – detergents, bleaches, disinfectants and household cleaners could make a lethal cocktail. The doctor often had the problem of determining what exactly the patient had swallowed, and how to treat them, as some of the would-be suicides were unconscious on arrival, and others were uncooperative.

Iron tablets were always a great temptation to children, as their shape and colour resembled certain types of popular sweets. They were also very dangerous when they were taken in excess, and after the stomach wash-out a clelate was also used as part of the treatment.

The local branch of the Samaritans occasionally brought patients in to Casualty who had taken overdoses. Included in this group were many of our regular clients who would take a few tables and then phone them for help. The more experienced members of that organisation knew them, and how to deal with them, but some of the newer members, showing great concern, would bring them in and stress their priority.

A sweet young lady Samaritan accompanied one such case while I was working on the desk one night.

'Please can you help this young lady?' she said. 'It's very urgent. She's taken an overdose of aspirin.'

I reached for a casualty card to fill in the details.

'Her name ...' she began.

'... is Mary Jones,' I replied.

'She lives at ...'

'Number 43 Dallas Drive,' I continued.

'She's aged 30.'

'No, she's 35.'

The good Samaritan looked at me.

'Oh, you know her?'

'We should do, this is the fifth time she's been in this month. We're old friends.'

'Is she likely to die?'

'I wouldn't think so, you must ask the staff, not me.'

I had a strong suspicion that their answer might be unrepeatable after so many wash-outs over the past month.

* * *

It was remarkable how the sight of a plastic tube, the stainless steel jugs and a nurse wearing a plastic apron had the effect of draining the courage of so-called tough men who had previously wanted to die. Andy was one such person. He was all muscle, and about six feet tall. After a quarrel with his girlfriend he had taken some paracetamol tablets, and then he promptly phoned her and told her what he had done, which resulted in his meeting with Millie, the staff nurse, and myself in the Gastric Lavage Room. I busied myself filling the metal jugs, while Millie donned her apron. Andy's eyes followed us all the time, and there were beads of perspiration on his brow. It wasn't until Millie broke the seal on the package containing the plastic tube and the syringe that he spoke.

'What's that for?' he enquired, eyeing the tube.

'I'm going to ask you to swallow it,' said Millie. 'If you do as I tell you, we'll soon get this business over and done with.'

'You're not sticking that thing down my throat.'

'It's absolutely essential that we wash out your stomach. The doctor did explain the reason why to you. It gives us no pleasure to do it, but those tablets have got to be removed.'

'You're not washing me out.'

Millie launched into the details once again of how and why it should be done, but Andy was adamant. He was going home and no one was going to wash his stomach out. Millie fetched the doctor, who again told him of the dangers of overdosing with paracetamol tablets, but it was to no avail.

'I'll give you an emetic then,' said the doctor.

'What's that?'

'Something to make you sick.'

'Sod off and leave me alone,' said Andy.

Millie followed the doctor outside the room, and I could hear a hum of conversation through the door. Andy sat up on the trolley.

'Get my clothes, I want to go home.'

'Wait a minute until the nurse comes back.'

It was nearer ten when Millie came bustling back. She was holding a piece of paper and a pen.

'Here you are, Andy,' she said. 'Sign this paper to say that you are taking your own discharge and refusing treatment.'

Andy swung from the trolley. 'What do you mean?'

'It relieves the hospital of any responsibility.'

'What responsibility?'

'Well, you could possibly die very soon after taking those tablets.'

'What?'

'We have been trying to get through to you how dangerous those tablets are. They will have an adverse effect on your liver, so there is nothing we can do about it. Your end will be quite a painful one.'

Andy for once was silent. Millie pressed on with a verbal barrage.

'Well come on, you told us to sod off. Now sign this form and you can sod off, I've got work to do. I want to help the people who want to live, not die.' And she gave me a wink from the head of the trolley.

'You are a bloody heartless bitch. I'm a patient here and I need attention.'

'When you refuse treatment there is nothing we can do.'

There was a long pause, and Andy's brain was working overtime.

'Will it hurt?' he finally asked.

'Not if you do as I tell you. But make up your mind, I've not got all day to piss about with you.'

There were no more protests from Andy. He lay on his side, the tube was inserted, and the washout was completed without any further trouble. He was removed from the Gastric Lavage Room and booked into a ward for observation and an overnight stay.

It was when I was clearing up afterwards that I had a chance to talk to Millie.

'You came down on him a bit hard, didn't you, Staff?'

'Not really. It usually works with that type of patient. It had to be done, although he wasn't a very pleasant character and I don't suppose we shall get any thanks for what we did. He could have died after swallowing such a large number of tablets.'

She gave me another wink as she went out the door.

* * *

The true intentions of any person attempting suicide can be assessed by their behaviour patterns. For the majority of patients who were admitted to Casualty, it was usually a cry for help to highlight problems such as failed love affairs, broken marriages and loneliness. People seriously intending to kill themselves work to a pre-arranged plan, quietly and efficiently, and leave nothing to chance.

The story of Tim's efforts to end his life were pieced together after the incident, and it would have made an excellent black comedy. Tim was one of life's dropouts. He was in his late twenties, unemployed and on his way to being an alcoholic. He was known to the members of our Casualty Department, owing to his frequent appearances after he'd been found in the city streets, collapsed through an overdose of alcohol.

He lived in a large rambling Victorian house in the red light area of the city. It was divided into bedsitting-rooms, and these were rented out mainly for the use of prostitutes as secondary accommodation for entertaining their clients. Tim had managed to rent the top-floor attic, probably because it was cheap. His room was sparsely furnished with a bed, a chair and an old set of drawers. The only daylight in the room was from an elevated glass panel in the roof.

In his efforts to leave what was for him a sorrowful world, Tim spent part of his unemployment cheque on a bottle of paracetamol and a bottle of whisky. He also acquired a length of rope from some undisclosed source, which according to the ambulance-men was rather thick and difficult to tie. He then wrote what was presumably meant to be his farewell letter, and in between drinking his neat whisky and taking the tablets, he tied one end of the rope to an overhead beam in the attic, and made a noose at the other. Finally he attempted to open his veins by cutting his wrists with a penknife, but only succeeded in causing surface lacerations. By this time he must have been very drunk and very weak, and with a final effort, he stood on the only chair in the room, put the noose round his neck and jumped.

The bedsitting-room directly under Tim's was occupied by a lady of the night who was entertaining a client at the time. If the ambulance-man's description of the event was correct, two naked bodies were locked together in heated passion. As they lay together, entwined in each other's arms, there was a tremendous crash from the attic above, and a shower of plaster and splintered wood rained down on them. When the dust in the room cleared, a man's foot could be seen protruding through a hole in the ceiling above them.

No one knew what really happened when Tim jumped off the chair. Perhaps the rope was badly tied, or it may have stretched. But one thing was certain: when his twelve stones of flesh hit the floor boards, the timber was so rotten and decayed by age and dampness that one foot went through the wood, hence through the ceiling of the room below, while the other landed on an intervening beam, leaving Tim suspended between Heaven and Hell.

In spite of the ensuing confusion, someone called an ambulance, and on its arrival Tim was found unconscious and lying in a pool of vomit, surrounded by a group of people discussing if it was necessary to give him the kiss of life. On observing the vomit, they must have had second thoughts, which was perhaps as well for Tim. As he was being carried down the stairs to the ambulance, on the floor below a man was seen struggling to put on a pair of trousers, at the same time demanding the return of his twenty pounds from a woman clad only in a dirty dressing gown.

I helped undress Tim on his arrival at the hospital. The smell of vomit and whisky still clung to his clothing. Being sick may have saved him from the effects of the tablets; the remains of them could be seen as he continued to heave and strain as he was turned on his side to prevent him from choking.

'He's going to have a hell of a hangover when he comes round,' Sister said.

'And a sore neck,' I said.

She directed her gaze at me.

'You, Mr Cockshaw, can help by getting a mop and bucket, and start removing this bloody mess off my floor while I fetch a doctor.'

I made a tactical withdrawal to the Utility Room while Tim, on cue, started to be sick again.

* * *

Of all the various ways of committing suicide, to immolate oneself by burning must be the worst. The few cases that came into the Casualty Department were nearly all from the Asian community, and although some were still alive when they were brought in, they died shortly afterwards. Soaking yourself in petrol or some other inflammable liquid and then igniting it reflects on a sorry state of mind.

Their reasons for doing it were varied. One girl was

concerned because she could not conceive, and was abused by her husband. Another was the victim of an arranged marriage to a man much older than herself who she had never met, and her parents were sending her to India for the ceremony. Mother-in-law problems were another reason for some Asian girls to terminate their lives, through the sheer unhappiness they suffered when they married and became a member of a new household. Perhaps it was a clash of cultures in some respect, and sadly these girls seemed to have no one to turn to for help. Had there been some organisation for the Asian community similar to our Samaritans, some of these victims might be alive today.

Those unsung stalwarts of the Ambulance Service, who had to go and pick up the pieces after some of these traumatic events, have an unenviable job. They have to remove the remains of suicides who have lain down on railway lines and been cut into sections by oncoming trains. They collect bodies from canals and rivers that may have been there for long periods. Guns are another means of terminating one's existence, leaving behind a gruesome mess.

A murder enquiry was once instigated by the police when they discovered a body in a burnt-out car in a lay-by, and found the cap from the petrol tank some distance away. It was only when they traced the victim, visited his house, and found suicide notes in his bedroom, that their suspicions were allayed. At the inquest it appeared that a broken love affair was the cause of the man's actions.

From the young girl of 14 who took an overdose after an abortion, to the old couple in their eighties who said they had nothing to live for, and made a suicide pact in which the wife died and the husband was found alive and brought into hospital, it is clear that these unhappy people are in no fit state of mind to realise the burden of suffering they leave behind for their families and friends. They also leave a sense of guilt with their loved ones that they were to blame in some way. They may wonder if perhaps had they been more aware and considerate, they might have prevented the last desperate act.

Alas, the clock cannot be put back, and in the final analysis, it is very doubtful if they could have changed the course of events.

Chapter 14

The Night the Sky Fell In

We are all deeply touched by certain events in our lives, and in spite of the passing years, they cannot be erased from our memories. As an outsider working in the Accident and Emergency Department, I can say that one incident occurred that had a profound effect on all the staff. That was the night the sky fell in.

It was a Sunday night, and considering it was January, the weather outside was dry and not too cold. The intake of patients for the night had been about average for this time of the year, and typical of the period between Christmas and Easter, when the weeks seemed to drag by. On Sunday night the Casualty Department always suffered from a shortage of pillows and blankets through excessive use over the weekend, and the porters always blamed the ambulance-men who, every time they brought a patient in, took a clean pillow and a clean blanket, leaving their dirty ones.

Fred the porter was changing the paper sheets on the trolley when the initial burst of activity happened. It was about half past eight; telephone bells started ringing and people started running. The flying squad ran to the storeroom and started donning their fluorescent jackets and checking their emergency packs. The Sister in charge started yelling for the porters.

'She's at it again, panic stations,' Fred was heard to mutter. 'Some silly bugger must have fallen off their bike outside Marks & Spencer's.' He walked slowly down the corridor towards her, and then came dashing back.

'Bloody hell, there's a plane crashed on the side of the motorway about twelve miles from here. Help me get as many trolleys as possible into the ambulance bay. The other porters are coming across to give us a hand.'

In a matter of minutes we had a line of eight trolleys standing in the bay. Some of the staff stood waiting, not knowing what to do, while on the reception desk the phones were ringing continuously, and the radio link with Ambulance Control was bellowing out instructions to the hospital and its vehicles. I looked round to see who needed any help.

'Is there anything I can do?' I asked Alf the reception clerk.

'I don't think so. I seem to be in the way here myself,' he said as he was pushed aside by one of the staff who grabbed at the phone on his desk.

It was an ironic situation, as every year around this time, the Emergency Services have a combined exercise to practise their procedures in case of a national disaster. The Ambulance Service, the Police, the Fire and Rescue Service, the St. John's Ambulance Service, the Red Cross and even the W.R.V.S. attended a fake accident scene to provide sustenance, in the way of food and drink. The patients for these exercises were volunteers from the Casualty Union, and they were made up according to the type of disaster that was being enacted. They were usually blooded up with a substance that looked like tomato sauce, and smothered in triangular bandages, and they lay on the ground feigning unconsciousness, or moaning and crying for help. Some of the exercises in the past had been simulated air disasters, and although it may have been good experience for those taking part, I got the impression that it was not taken very seriously by the majority of the participants.

Over the years, the Accident and Emergency Department had been put on red alert by our local airport whenever any incoming plane got into difficulty through engine trouble or faulty landing gear; but fortunately there had never been any major incident and the full emergency services had never swung into action. But tonight was the real thing, and I wondered how the hospital would cope with the situation. I was soon to find out.

During the next half hour, activity in the department increased, and the story of the crash gradually unfolded via national and local radio. The plane had left Heathrow Airport on a flight to Belfast, and just after take-off the pilot had reported that one of his engines was on fire, and he was going to land at a local airport. Sadly, it was not to be. Just in sight of the runway, and with only under a mile to go, the plane skimmed over the rooftops of a village on one side of the busy motorway, and struck the embankment on the other side, breaking up into sections. Some of the wreckage was strewn over the motorway, and it was a miracle how the high speed traffic managed to avoid it. If it hadn't, the casualties would have been even more numerous.

There were now ambulances and medical flying squads from three Midland hospitals. Reports of the number of fatalities ranged wildly from fifty to one hundred, as at that early stage no one quite knew the number of people who were trapped inside the plane. By some miracle it did not catch fire, and the Fire Brigade, who were at the scene within minutes, helped to reduce the threat by using foam to combat any possibility of a blaze. As news of the crash spread, the Casualty staff increased dramatically. Doctors, surgeons, nurses, porters and administrators seemed to arrive from out of the woodwork. The existing patients were ushered home if possible, or sent to the wards, and then to my amazement, the waiting room doors were locked and the lights put out, so that the hospital could deal solely with the crash victims. It must have been the first time in the history of the hospital that this had ever happened. From the earliest date of its opening in 1771, it had advertised that it was open for "the sick, lame and poor of any county or nation". Perhaps the events of that night determined the actions of the staff; but I wondered if it was right. After all, the local people would still need some medical cover, as there was no other accident and emergency department in the city. I was to confront this problem later.

Within the next hour there were so many people in the department that it was difficult to determine who was in charge. Voices were raised, and orders were issued. The staff were reinforced by more doctors and nurses from the wards, and staff were being called from their homes. I even noticed two clergymen hovering in the background, and for the first time since I had worked in the department, I felt that I was in the way. My thoughts flew back to Mrs Pushbutton at the W.R.V.S, who had been involved in training for such an emergency many years ago, and I wondered how she must be feeling now. This was for real, and I hoped that any training from the past would be of good use tonight.

Sadly, I decided to go home. I had worked in the department for a long time and helped with many traumatic incidents, but now the professionals had completely taken over, which was their right, and I was no longer needed.

I made my way from Casualty to the main foyer, to the reception desk to pick up my coat. To my surprise the area was crowded. Myrtle, the night receptionist for the main complex, was besieged by a mass of humanity round her counter, and both her phones were ringing as she struggled to answer them. At the same time, she beckoned to me to join her, so I pushed my way through the door and went behind the desk.

'What's going on?' I enquired.

She gave a shrug of her shoulders.

'No one has bothered to inform me about the air crash,' she replied. 'The first thing I knew about it was when this stream of patients started coming in the main foyer because Casualty was closed to them. I'm trying to get some help.'

'Can I give you a hand?'

'I wish you would, Walter.'

All the patients were sitting on chairs opposite the reception desk, apart from one lady in a wheelchair, and it was mostly their relations that surrounded the counter, seeking attention for their sick and injured. They were confused by the whole situation, and obviously they had no knowledge of the plane crash, as they were demanding to know why the Casualty Department was closed.

Myrtle, with her big eyes and lovely long hair, was taking it all in her stride, cool and efficient as ever. She started to explain that there was an emergency at the hospital, and if they would be patient she would try and get a doctor to see them as soon as possible. Her calmness had a reassuring effect; she had that certain quality in dealing with people.

'Take over the desk, Walter, I'll try and get a member of the Casualty staff to come and help.'

The relatives moved from the counter and then the phones started to ring again. It has always amazed me how fast bad news travels. Most of the callers were seeking information that I could not give them, and then I realised that, for a few giddy minutes, I was in sole charge of what was now the remains of the Accident and Emergency Department. Mrs. Pushbutton would have been proud of me.

The news on the radio brought enquiries from the local population, asking if they could give blood if it was needed, and although I knew it would not be necessary, I took their names and telephone numbers. A young girl arrived accompanied by her father. She had been bitten by a dog and had a small laceration on her hand. I suggested that she should visit her G.P. in the morning rather than wait indefinitely at the hospital; the father seemed satisfied after being informed of the situation. Another worried mother sat nursing her young daughter who had a needle sticking through her foot. I kept going over to her and reassuring the child that we would get a doctor to see her as soon as possible.

After some time, Myrtle reappeared on the scene.

'Any luck?' I asked.

'None of the doctors want to come,' she replied. 'But I've brought some casualty cards. At least we can book the patients in. We can't use the computer so we shall have to write them by hand. Can you fetch me a trolley, there's a patient we shall have to send to the ward as she's had a miscarriage. I'll try and arrange it.'

I fetched the trolley from Casualty, and discovered the staff still gathered in groups, waiting for any casualties that might be on their way. In the meantime, Myrtle had arranged with the Gynaecology Unit to accept the lady who had miscarried, so I wheeled her to the ward.

On my return I went round booking in the rest of the patients. There were none that required immediate attention, they were all walking wounded, but some with possible bone injuries would no doubt need an X-ray. Strangely enough, no one seemed to mind waiting, and I had the impression that they were more interested in what was happening at the hospital than in their own problems.

The news from the site of the crash continued to filter through, and the latest estimate of the number of people killed was now 50. The hospital had sent a number of its staff to the crash site, along with the necessary life support systems. The press, never far from the scene of any disaster, descended like vultures on the hospital. First came the reporters from the local newspapers and radio stations, followed by the national press and the television crews with all their equipment. All of them asked questions and got no answers from our desk. We were besieged, and it was only after Myrtle phoned the administration officer for advice, that it was decided to open the board room as a press office. As this was on the far side of the hospital, I had to escort them through the underground passages and along the corridors. It was a continuous job throughout the night.

Patients were still arriving at the main reception desk, some by car and some by ambulance. No doctor had come to see them yet. Myrtle once again disappeared in the direction of Casualty to try and get some medical help – without success, as the first casualties had now started to come in from the crash. We continued to fill in casualty cards for the new arrivals in between answering the phone and dealing with the press. Through the doors also came deliveries of blankets, probably from some of the other local hospitals, and it was sad to think that it took an air disaster to produce clean linen for the hospital on Sunday nights.

As no doctor had come yet to check the patients waiting in the main foyer, Myrtle was getting concerned. It was then that the overdose arrived. It is an amazing fact that when the Casualty staff were working at full stretch, an overdose patient invariably arrived on the scene. Perhaps this was the turning point in our situation, as Myrtle once again went in search of a doctor, this time with positive results.

'The doctor's agreed to see the patients in the Fracture Clinic, Walter, so we can take the patients round there.' There was a note of relief in her voice.

Like good shepherds, we took our sheep round to the Fracture Clinic and handed them over to the staff who had been brought in for the emergency, and so far had not received any patients to deal with. I think they were glad to have some work to do while they were waiting.

News from the scene of the crash came from various sources as the night passed, most of it contradictory, and the reported numbers of the dead and injured continued to vary. The police had now opened a Control Room in the hospital, and B.B.C. radio programmes were broadcasting emergency telephone numbers for anxious relatives to ring for any available information about the passengers, as the dead and injured were being taken to two other Midland hospitals besides our own. It was a confusing situation, and identification and whereabouts of some of the victims was proving to be difficult.

The main reception desk in the foyer remained a focal point for most of the enquiries, as the Casualty Department was by this time receiving patients from the crash. Sadly, relatives of the passengers started arriving at the hospital after travelling through the night to discover the fate of their loved ones, only to discover that they might have come to the wrong hospital. They were under the impression that as the plane had crashed within our county boundary, the victims must all have been brought to the local hospital. Even if we had known their fate, we could not have passed the knowledge on, as this was the duty of the police and the staff. All we could do was refer them to these authorities. It must have been an agonising time for them as they waited, and Myrtle, with her sympathy and understanding, was again an angel in disguise. She tried to allay everyone's fears with reassurance and cups of tea, and made constant enquiries to the Control Room on their behalf

It was about three o'clock on the Monday morning when the last victim in the plane was released, and the full extent of the tragedy could be assessed. The press and the television crews were as active as ever, and it was only when I left for home that the full impact of the disaster hit me. In a minor way I had been involved, and although I had not been on the scene of the crash helping the injured, I had been on the inside looking in at what I hoped would be my last experience of a plane crash.

The morning newspapers had banner headlines about the incident, and the television reports showed the harrowing scenes. There were many heroic deeds performed by people on the spot when the crash occurred. Drivers on the motorway and residents from the nearby village went to assist the victims. Some of the passengers from the plane miraculously escaped unhurt and suffered only from shock; but many remained trapped inside the wreck, badly injured or dead. The medical teams worked throughout the night with the Police, the Fire Service, and the Ambulance Service. The nurses from the flying squad from the Accident and Emergency Department, many of them quite young, and who had never before been involved in such a traumatic event, worked hand-in-hand with the doctors and surgeons. My friend Mike, the orthopaedic surgeon, had to climb into the wrecked body of the plane and carry out some amputations.

The pilot, suffering from multiple injuries, was among the patients brought back to the hospital, and it was only much later that the people in the nearby village realised how much they owed to his skill in avoiding the populated area where they lived. At least 46 people died that night, and a great many were injured. The motorway was closed for three days while the wreckage was removed from the scene, and the area cleared.

It was impossible to estimate how much human misery and unhappiness resulted from the crash. The losses were great, and the people who died left gaps in the lives of those they left behind that would never be filled.

Perhaps some day the full story of the incident will be written in terms of human endeavour. If so, I hope that many people like golden-haired Myrtle, whose work and compassion also helped, will not be forgotten.

There must be many lessons to be learnt by the Emergency Services from this incident. Although there was an official enquiry, it was sad that the scope of the investigation was not widened to take in the opinions of some of the observers. It is easy to be wise after such a disaster, but when the sky does fall in, we must be ready for such an event.

Chapter 15

Christmas. The Nurse's Lament

A Merry Christmas in the Cas. Who said that? they must be mad.
Far away from the season's glee, poor working nurses just like me.
Tend the drunks, and make the tea, and never once do we stop running.
'... Alright Dear, your bedpan's coming ...'

It was the Festive season again. Christmas, followed by the New Year, was always one of the busiest times for the staff in the Casualty Department, mainly through over indulgence of eating and drinking. During this period there was a great influx of patients, and the waiting room was always full. It was a season of remembrance too, a recalling of memories of loved ones from the past, a time of nostalgia as well as good will. Violence also overshadowed the event due to excessive drinking, and the celebrations encompassed the whole spectrum of human behaviour.

The spirit of good will pervaded the hospital. Dozens of Christmas cards were exchanged between members of the staff, and the children's wards were overwhelmed by gifts and toys. I was always surprised by the kind but rather misplaced charity of the people of the city, who went to such great efforts to buy or collect toys for the children who had to stay in hospital. It was an embarrassment to receive so many, as it was the hospital's policy to discharge as many of their young patients as possible to spend Christmas with their own families, and the children that were left behind were usually too ill to bother with the toys. It was a pity such kindness could not have been directed into other channels, as there were many old people without any families who would have loved someone to visit them, and to receive a gift.

It was early on Christmas Eve when I stepped out of my car, and a bitter wind swept over the open courtyard. I could see the lights of the Christmas tree through the frosted window, and marvelled at the fact that it was still intact; it had been there now for nearly a week without being vandalised by some drunken patient. I pushed my way through the door and stopped at the reception desk. Debbie looked up from her book as I entered.

'Busy?' I asked.

'Take a look in there,' she said, pointing in the general direction of the waiting room.

But there was no need for me to look. I could guess by the volume of noise that was coming from inside that the room was full. I stopped, however, and opened the door to gaze inside. It was seething with bodies. I noticed Helen, obviously homeless again, surrounded by her Guinness bottles and plastic bags. Paddy Murphy and Billy Button were kicking hell out of the tea machine. Mixed groups of teenagers, some with tinsel in their hair, were singing and laughing. A young girl was being sick in a newspaper, and her boyfriend was trying to comfort her. Frightened small children huddled close to their parents. This mixture of singing, yelling, cursing and moaning mass of humanity contributed to a grand cacophony of sound that could only mean it was Christmas Eve again. Good will to all men.

I made my way to the staff room. Some unwashed cups stood on a small table; this was always an indication that the department was working in top gear. From underneath the piles of clothes and scarves hanging on the hooks, I managed to extract a white coat that had been deposited by one of the doctors. It was far too large, but it was the only one available so it would have to do. I put it on, went into the corridor and found Danny the shift leader, who was in charge of the porters.

'I'm glad to see you,' he said. 'My shift has not had a break since they came on duty.'

'Where do you want me?'

'Give a hand here, then I can go for a cup of tea.' Without giving me a chance to answer, he made his way to the Porters' Lodge.

Ken came out of the Resuscitation Room carrying an oxygen cylinder as the noise from the waiting room echoed along the corridor and changed into a song, with uplifted voices giving a rendition of "Why are we waiting?" This wave of sound carried past the cubicles and into the treatment area. There was a look of disgust on Ken's face.

'Listen to those drunken sods, half of them are from parties, and they've been here all afternoon. They've pissed up and they expect us to give them priority over the genuine patients. The poor bugger in there,' he went on, pointing in the direction of the Resuscitation Room, 'has had one arrest and is in a bad way. I don't think he'll make it. His wife is in Sister's office.'

'I suppose it's all part of life's rich pattern, Ken.'

'I get fed up with this job at Christmas. I'm not paid to fight and argue with drunks suffering from self-inflicted injuries. By the way, there's a washout to be done. Will you help Millie?'

For most people, Christmas is a time of good will with a religious message, but for some individuals – the old, the lonely and the unwanted – the message is different. They feel cut off and isolated, and it is then their despair often takes the extreme form of suicide attempts.

It was strange how incidents always came in cycles, particularly stomach wash-outs. Watching the contents of a patient's stomach slowly reappear along a clear plastic tube before they drained into a bucket at the side of the trolley was no aid to one's appetite, and tonight, after the third washout, the food on the menu in the dining hall lost its appeal. I had no desire for Christmas pudding or chips.

The ever changing scene in any casualty department involving patients and staff who are linked together, even for a short period, adds to the understanding and experience of both parties. As I left the Resuscitation Room after helping with the last stomach washout, the doors of the ambulance bay swung open, and Michael, the officer from the Ambulance Control, came in blowing his cupped hands as if to warm them.

'A Merry Christmas, Mike. What brings you out of your Ivory Tower?'

'Shortage of staff, pissed up people, and bloody idiots having accidents through celebrating too early.'

'I'm sorry your celebrations have been spoilt. I'll lock the doors and put the closed notice up if you want me to.'

'I wish you would. Can you find me a trolley? I've got a patient waiting in the cold outside.'

It took me about five minutes to find one. There was a line of trolleys, all occupied, that stretched the whole length of the corridor, and there was still a queue at the reception desk waiting to be booked in. I began to wonder how the staff were going to cope.

Weaving my way past the waiting column, and trying to avoid a pool of vomit on the floor, I pushed the trolley to where Michael stood waiting.

'Here you are, Michael, I'll collect my Christmas present later. Do you want a hand with your patient?'

'It might be as well, I think she may have broken her leg.'

'Is she one of your pissed up patients, or one of the bloody idiots who has been celebrating too early?'

'Neither.'

'What happened to her then?'

'She fell of the back of an elephant.'

The noise from the waiting room reached a new crescendo as a fresh rendering of "Silent Night" echoed along the corridor, making normal conversation difficult. I turned to Michael once again and yelled at him.

'Sorry about the noise. I thought you said that the patient had fallen from an elephant.'

'I did... She has... So let's get her inside where it's warm, or I shall be here all night.'

We moved outside to the back of the ambulance, and with the help of the other member of the crew, we lifted the canvas sheet between us that the patient was lying on, and managed to transfer her on to the trolley and into the department. It was then I noticed the patient's costume before she was covered with a blanket. It was an off-the-shoulder red dress that finished just below her thighs, and she wore a matching pair of tights. Both the dress and the tights were decorated with sequins that sparkled under the fluorescent light, but her left leg had been encased in a temporary splint. I thought it prudent to make sure that the blanket covered her up to her chin, to avoid any comments from the passing drunks. She gave a little groan as we tried to make her more comfortable, and then she was put in line with the other patients.

Once again I turned to Michael.

'Who is she?'

'Sabrina, the Elephant Woman.'

'You're joking.'

'I'm not. She's with the circus at the Granby Halls, and she's had a fall off the back of her jumbo during a rehearsal. Can you get her booked in, and let us get out of this madhouse.'

Sabrina the Elephant Woman turned out to be Ethel Ramsden from Yorkshire, and her details were formally recorded. As I added her casualty card to the pile, Sister stopped me and looked over my shoulder.

'What's happened to this lady?', she enquired.

'A leg injury, Sister.'

'Another traffic accident?'

'In a way. She fell off an elephant.'

She paused and gave me a long hard look.

'A bloody pink one, I suppose,' she said before hurrying off along the corridor.

* * *

A Merry Christmas in the Cas. Who said that? They must be mad.
The Sister's in a foul mood, she's missed her sleep she's missed her food.
The porters all have disappeared, the X-rays lie forgotten ...
'... Oh can't you take your own socks off? Your feet smell something rotten.'

* * *

It was cold in the ambulance bay; the December wind seemed to penetrate through our clothing in spite of the warm air that was circulating from an overhead fan heater. The staff nurse, who was wrapped in her cloak, stood shivering and the porter who was also at hand stood stamping his feet on the concrete as if he was participating in some ritual dance.

'This sounds like the ambulance,' said the nurse as the distant sound of a siren could be heard. 'Tell the doctor the patient is here.'

If the trimmings and tinsel that obscure the face of Christmas were torn away, they would reveal the heartbreak and tragedy that existed alongside the festivities. It was strange how one simple telephone call could alter the pace of the department, by alerting the staff and redirecting their efforts. In this case it was from Ambulance Control to say that an unconscious young male patient was on his way with breathing difficulties. As it was never easy for the medical staff to predict the condition of any patient before arrival, both the doctor and Sister stood outside waiting for the ambulance.

Before the vehicle had even stopped, the porter had opened the rear doors to reveal an ambulance-man bending over a still form inside. He stood up as the doctor and Sister entered. His face looked ashen under the pale white light. He shrugged his shoulders as he turned to them.

'I'm sorry, I did my best for him,' he said. 'I think he's gone. There was no pulse when we arrived at the scene, and we were there in minutes after receiving the call.'

'What happened?' asked the doctor as he bent over the patient, checking with his stethoscope.

'His parents had gone out, and he was having a party at home with some of his school friends. Apparently he was drinking his father's whisky; he drank about two thirds of a bottle, so I'm told.'

'How old was he?'

'About 15. His friends were drinking beer and cider, and they got worried when he was violently sick and started choking. They fetched a neighbour, who dialled for an ambulance when he noticed the lad wasn't breathing properly.'

'Have the parents been notified?' Sister asked.

'The police are trying to get in touch with them.'

The doctor finished his examination, and put his stethoscope back in his pocket. He climbed out of the ambulance and shook his head.

'I'm sorry, there's nothing I can do for the lad,' he said. 'He's another victim of the demon drink.'

It was an hour later when the mortal remains of George were wheeled into a side room off the main corridor to await formal identification by his parents, who were now on their way in a police car. Sister thought that it would have added to their distress to make the journey across a dimly lit court-yard to the cold grey confines of the Winter Gardens to complete their grim task.

'Stay with him, Walter, until his parents arrive,' she said. 'I don't want any of those stupid drunks wandering in here, they are crawling all over the place as it is.'

And so I was left to keep vigil over George. As I pulled back the sheet that covered his face, I could smell the mixture of whisky and vomit that still clung to him in spite of the efforts of the staff to make him more presentable. As I gazed down at him, I saw his face had now relaxed to a more peaceful expression from the twisted look that it had worn when he was brought in. With his appearance of youth and innocence, it was hard to realise he was locked in eternal sleep. There was no tomorrow for him. His Christmas gifts would remain unopened, his words of thanks unspoken, and his family would die a little with his passing.

The noise from the waiting room came in waves and permeated through the closed door. Half sung carols, mixed with yells and screams and burst of laughter reached my ears, and I covered George's face again as if to protect him from the mingled sounds outside. I even wondered if he would sleep quieter when he was taken down to the Winter Gardens. It seemed to be an affront to human dignity for him to be subjected to the rowdy behaviour of the people in the waiting room.

The click of the door made me look up and focus my thoughts as the nurse whispered, 'They're here now.'

Sister entered first, followed by a man with his arm round

the shoulders of a woman, as if to support her. He paused just inside the doorway and turned to her. 'Are you sure?' he asked in a voice that trembled with emotion.

She answered by nodding her head, but her whole frame was shaking, and the tears that were running down her face had left lines on her carefully applied make-up. Her perfume mingled with the hospital odours in the room. The evening shawl round her shoulders and the short black cocktail dress with the red corsage seemed strangely out of place in the charged atmosphere. The parents moved forward to the trolley, and as I stood back, Sister lifted the sheet from the lad's face. The woman gave a choking cry and moved forward, clutching her son to her breast. She rocked to and fro, her cries reverberating round the room. The impact of her loss had penetrated that shield of courage she had used as a barrier when she had first entered the room.

I eased my way to the door, and Sister nodded to me as a sign of dismissal. As I stepped outside, the wave of sound in the corridor reached a new peak, the voices uplifted in song rang out from the waiting room.

'...We wish you a merry Christmas ... We wish you a merry Christmas ... We wish you a merry Christmas and a happy New Year ...'

* * *

A Merry Christmas in the Cas. Who said that?
They must be mad.
Every minute, every hour, our work is never done.
Giving people injections is never really fun.
'... Where do you want the needle, in your arm or
in your bum ...?'

* * *

The clock registered 20 minutes after midnight, and I pushed yet another patient along the corridor to join the queue at the X-ray Department. The man on the trolley groaned at the sight of the milling crowd.

'Bloody hell, I shall be here until next Christmas, judging by this lot in front of me.'

'Serves you right,' said his female companion. 'You should stay off the booze.'

As I picked up the X-ray form to hand it to the radiographer he caught my arm.

'Where can I buy some fags?' he asked. 'I've got to have a smoke.'

'Nowhere here,' I replied.

'Do you have a machine or a shop?'

'No.'

'Does your dining room sell them?'

'No, this is a hospital.'

'So what..?'

'We don't allow smoking, we don't encourage patients to die of cancer.'

A barrage of curses followed me into the X-ray Department and Anne, who was on duty, gave me a smile.

'Was he trying to tell you that your parents weren't married, Walter?'

'Something like that.'

As I put the form on the desk, there was a sudden uproar from the next room, and a woman's voice that I recognised as Claudia's, one of the radiographers, was raised in outrage. I dashed inside. A man was lying on a trolley clutching a sprig of mistletoe, the blanket that should have been covering him was now on the floor, and he was exposing far more of his body that was decent. Claudia was standing in the corner of the room looking tense, her body stiff and her fists clenched.

'What the hell's going on?' I asked.

'Salright,' said the man on the trolley in a slurred voice. 'It's Christmas. I'm trying to make everyone happy.'

'That doesn't mean that you can put your hand up my skirt, you dirty bugger,' said Claudia.

'My hand slipped.'

'If it slips again you will be off that bloody trolley and outside. Put him in the corridor, Walter, and stay with him while I bring his plates.'

I pushed him outside and past the other waiting patients while his X-rays were being processed. The man I had brought down previously was trying to borrow a cigarette from a patient in front of him, and his female companion started battering him on the head with her handbag as he tried to get down of his trolley. Meanwhile, the Mistletoe Man started shouting at two passing nurses, and extended an invitation for them to come and join him on his trolley, and have a good time.

'If you don't behave I'll have to put you outside.'

'I want to have a piss.'

'Wait until you get back to Casualty.'

'I can't wait.'

'You shouldn't drink so much.'

I stayed with him until his X-ray plates were ready, and returned him to the treatment area. I found a cubicle empty, so I put him inside and pulled the curtains round him.

'Stay there and don't move while I get you a bottle.'

Passing the patients now crowding the corridor, and trying to avoid a pool of vomit, I made my way to the sluice room to get a bottle. Running the gauntlet of enquiries about ambulances to take patients back home, requests for cups of tea and "could a relative have an aspirin tablet for a headache", I finally got back to the cubicle with the bottle for the Mistletoe Man.

It was a journey in vain. As I approached, Sister pulled back the curtains round the cubicle to reveal him standing in all his glory, holding his hand on the wall to steady himself, while he urinated into the wash-hand basin. I waited for the explosion from Sister, and it wasn't long in coming.

'You dirty filthy bugger, you are not fit to associate with decent people. You go out and get drunk, and we are expected not only to treat your injuries, but also clean your filth up afterwards, all at the expense of genuine patients who really need our help. Your X-rays are alright, you haven't broken any bones, but you had better piss off before I break your bloody neck. Help him get dressed, Walter, and get rid of him.' She turned away in disgust.

I escorted the Mistletoe Man outside when he was dressed, and the last I saw of him was when he was trying to kiss a policewoman, who was not enjoying the experience, by the look on her face.

* * *

A Merry Christmas in the Cas. Who said that? They must be mad.
No "Shepherds Watch" no "Silent Night, no carols to set the scene.
Only a drunk in the waiting room who's singing about Nellie Dean.
I wish I'd taken Mum's advice and married someone rich and nice.
No more days and no more nights ... 'Oh don't be sick all down my tights.'

* * *

Polly, a young student nurse, looked decidedly unhappy as she tried her best to perform her duties. After all, it was Christmas, and six successive nights on duty, as well as three large glasses of wine forced on her by her friends before she started work, had taken their toll. Polly did not usually drink alcohol, but she had given way on this occasion, as it was the festive season. She was now regretting it.

Sister was well aware of her condition. It wasn't that Polly was drunk, it was the ill effects from the wine. When she saw the young nurse make a sudden dash to the toilet to be sick, she decided that Polly should take a rest somewhere.

So I was called in to help carry her from the staff toilet, where she had fainted.

'Where can we put her, Sister?' I enquired.

'Put her on a bed in the Casualty Ward, and ask the staff nurse to keep an eye on her,' she replied.

With some assistance from the porters, Polly was duly deposited on the only spare bed that was available, which happened to be in the men's section, and the curtains were drawn round her. Polly was obviously out of action for the rest of the night, and for a time it was a case of out of sight, out of mind. That was, until the chief nursing officer appeared on the scene.

The chief nursing officer was a very nice person, but she was also a very strict disciplinarian, and it was her habit to make occasional visits to the Casualty Department at night. Her main intention on this occasion must have been to wish everyone a Happy Christmas, but that didn't mean she would overlook any misbehaviour on the part of any member of the staff under her care.

With Polly evidently in mind, Sister stopped me as I passed by. 'Go and warn the nurse on the Casualty Ward that the chief nursing officer is in the department, just in case she goes in there to pay a visit.'

Mo the staff nurse was missing when I entered, and it was a few minutes before she returned.

'Where have you been, Mo? Sister has sent me to tell

you that the chief nursing officer is doing her rounds. She might be coming in here.'

'Well, I'm not Superwoman. Even I go for a pee now and again. I'm not likely to get a break tonight with that lot out there.' She gestured in the direction of the waiting room.

She had hardly finished speaking when the chief nursing officer walked in. After exchanging seasonable greetings, she looked round the ward.

'I see you are full up tonight.'

'Yes,' said Mo.

'I'll just have a check on the patients,' she said.

She moved to the first bed. 'Who's this patient?' she asked.

'Oh, it's Mr. Jones, a head injury.'

Mo gave her a description of the symptoms of the other four patients who were being kept in for overnight observation. It was then that the chief nursing officer stopped at the curtained-off bed where Polly was sleeping.

'Oh, in there..?'

'Yes.'

'Er ... That's Mr. Smith. He's on a bedpan at the moment.' Mo had her fingers crossed as she spoke. 'It's another head injury.'

'I'd better not look then, I don't want to embarrass him,' the chief nursing officer said with a smile. 'A Happy Christmas to you both.' She walked to the door and turned.

'By the way, your Mr. Smith wears expensive perfume,' she said.

* * *

Ron the reception clerk waved urgently as I passed him in the corridor. He was filling in an admission form for a patient who was waiting for removal to a ward.

'For Heaven's sake, Walter, give me a hand, there's a whole queue of people waiting to be booked in at the desk. I've got a feeling that there's going to be a riot in the waiting room soon.'

He was not far wrong. Both the telephones were ringing, and one of the nurses was trying to explain to a patient who had just arrived, and was obviously drunk, that he could not receive priority treatment for his cut hand, just because he had a sister who worked in the hospital kitchens.

I picked up the nearest phone to answer it.

'Accident and Emergency Department.'

'Is that the Casualty?'

'Yes.'

'Can I talk to the dentist?'

'What dentist?'

'The one on duty.'

'We don't have one on duty.'

'You must have. Every hospital has a dentist.'

'I'm sorry, it's now Christmas Day, and our dental surgeon is only on call for very serious facial injuries. Why do you ask?'

'My husband's been suffering from chronic toothache for two weeks now, and he wants a tooth extracting.'

'Why tonight?'

'It's going to spoil his Christmas.'

'I can give you the phone number of an emergency dentist. You can contact him on Boxing Day.'

'He's been paying his National Health for years. We have no transport. Can you send an ambulance for him?'

'I'm sorry, I can't do that ...'

I withdrew the phone about six inches from my ear as a tirade of four-letter curses came from the disgruntled lady at the other end of the line. She had obviously been drinking. As I waited, there was a scream from the corner of the waiting room as two male figures started aiming blows at each other. A burly police constable who happened to be on the scene hurried across, grabbed a collar in each hand and pulled them apart. The woman at the other end of the phone was running out of swear words, and I thought it was time to intervene.

'Madam, do you want the details of the emergency dentist?'

She obviously did not by her answer, and it was a physical impossibility to respond to her suggestion of what I could do with this particular gentleman. I turned to the next person in the queue. He was carrying a small girl.

'Can I help you, Sir?'

'It's my daughter. Anticipating the visit of Father Christmas, she woke up early and started playing with her toys, and now she's got a piece of Lego stuck up her nose.'

The little girl, frightened by all the noise and the drunken behaviour of the crowd in the waiting room, clung to her father. I beckoned them through the door, found them a quiet seat in the main corridor out of the way and hurried back to answer the ever ringing phone, again with the stock enquiry.

'Accident and Emergency. Can I help you?'

There was a rush of words. 'You should have a Mr. Smith in your waiting room. No doubt he has that old bag with him again. Would you tell him that he can go and sleep at his mother's house tonight as I'm locking all the doors and going to bed.'

The phone was slammed down at the other end before I could reply. I replaced the receiver and went out into the waiting room and shouted, 'Is there a Mr. Smith here, please?' My voice hardly penetrated through the noise. So I tried again with double the volume. 'IS THERE A MR. SMITH HERE, PLEASE?' To my amazement everyone stopped talking and there was complete silence as three men emerged from the crowd and made their way towards me. The youngest man was about twenty, the other two must have been in their thirties, and they were all accompanied by members of the opposite sex. Somewhat bewildered I asked.

'Are you all named Smith?'

They looked at each other and paused, then they nodded their heads in unison. I looked at the three females and tried to determine which one was the old bag.

'I have a message for Mr. Smith from a lady who did not leave her address, and she suggests that the Mr. Smith concerned should sleep at his mother's house tonight, as she's locking him out and going to bed.'

As I walked away, they all stood looking at each other, and I wondered if there would be three erring sons returning to their mother's arms that Christmas morning.

* * *

A Merry Christmas in the Cas. Who said that?
They must be mad.
I'm tired of paying for that Doctor's beer. I know
his pay cheque won't be here.
But his eyes are kind, and they glow so red every
time I mention bed.
Stomach wash-outs by the score, and vomit bowls
galore.
I've changed my knickers twice tonight and I
haven't more.

* * *

The queue at the reception desk lengthened, and the atmosphere in the waiting room got more tense. I was glad that the glass partition separated us from the waiting patients and their friends and relatives who flooded the area. The glass panels above the counter reverberated from the fists of some of the angry patients as they hammered away at them. Almost everyone we had booked in seemed to be demanding priority treatment. Cynthia the staff nurse was trying her best to categorise the patients according to the seriousness of their illnesses or injuries, but she was finding it difficult to explain to the waiting crowd why a man with a head injury who had just arrived was next on the list for treatment.

'My husband has been here for two hours,' screamed one woman. 'Are you going to let him bleed to death?' She moved across the room, holding the wall to steady herself.

'I've checked his cut hand, and he will be alright for the time being,' said the staff nurse.

'We shall be here until next bloody Christmas if you don't get your finger out,' the woman replied, and without waiting for a response, she took a swing at Cynthia with her handbag. Fortunately, owing to her inebriated state, the blow missed, and from that point onwards any good relations that existed between the patients and staff deteriorated rapidly. Cynthia retreated to the door leading to the corridor, followed by the woman, who was still shouting abuse at her. I left the desk to try and help her, but two policemen waiting in the department, hearing the commotion, arrived on the scene at the same time. It was impossible to calm the drunken female, who was now swinging her handbag blindly at anyone who approached her.

'Can't you get her treated and get rid of her?' one of the policemen asked.

'She's not here to be treated.'

'What's she here for?'

'She's here with her husband who's cut his hand on a beer bottle and he's waiting to be seen. We have more serious cases to attend to at the moment.'

'Alright, leave it to us,' the policeman replied, and nodding to his companion, they advanced on the woman. I moved back behind the counter and the safety of the glass screen.

The Great British Public love to watch free live spectacles, providing that they do not have to participate in them. Perhaps they have been weaned on a diet of television violence over the years. The two policemen lifted the still screaming woman away from the corridor door and back into the waiting room, and the noise level there subsided considerably as "Silent Night" and "Come All Ye Faithful" died away and were replaced by three upraised voices yelling at the same time.

'Take your hands off her, you bastards!'

'Leave her alone, you pigs!'

'That's my mother, you pair of sods.'

I was never sure who started throwing things as it happened so suddenly, but Ron was already phoning for the porters for help, and for police reinforcements. The mini-riot that ensued only appeared to involve the woman's relatives, but while it lasted it was an uproarious affair. What a pity John Wayne wasn't around to see it! The non-participants gathered at one side of the waiting room and watched with great interest as the porters and the police struggled with six members of the same family on the other side. It was noticeable that not one of the onlookers offered to help as the tide of battle turned against the two policemen and the staff, and even Ron and I were about to shed our coward's cloaks and join in to help when some flashing blue lights could be seen through the waiting room window. Like the end of every good western, the American cavalry arrived just in time in the guise of four hefty policemen.

The action carried on for some time afterwards, and in spite of the offenders being handcuffed, it did not stop them lashing out with their feet before they were dragged outside to the waiting police cars, with the exception of the man with the cut hand, who was left behind for treatment, accompanied by a policeman.

Over the next two hours the crowd in the waiting room thinned slightly, and the domestic staff arrived with their mops and buckets to clean the area before going home to join their own families for Christmas. They prodded the inert bodies of the sleeping drunks, and made them move over so that they could clear the mess and the pools of vomit that were left in the corners of the room. The tramps who had come in from out of the cold and knew the routine, moved without being asked, and curled up again in the clean area, safe in the knowledge that they would probably be undisturbed by the staff; after all, it was Christmas.

I looked at my watch. It was nearly five o'clock, and I visualised the thousands of small children waking up to the thrill of another Christmas Day. Throwing off the mantle of sleep, they would have started to explore the presents that Santa Claus had left behind. But for some families, the day would be overcast with sorrow, with no guiding star to show them the way.

* * *

A Merry Christmas in the Cas. Who said that? They must be mad.
With so much work I feel so blue, can't make my date can't make the loo.
So I'll cross my legs and carry on, my bladder is weak but my spirit is strong.
'... What's that Sister ... What did you say, stop and have a drink?'

My God, she's human after all. A thought I'd never think.
'Yes, I'll have another pie, and one more gin and tonic.
... Doctor, take your hand away. You know I'm not bionic.

* * *

Dave the porter came bursting through the reception door, and Ron turned to greet him.

'If you want a drink it'll have to be coffee, the tea-bags have all gone.'

'I'm taking over. Sister wants you both to join her in her office. She's got some food and drink waiting, so push off.'

Dave was like that, brusque and straight to the point.

Sister's office was crowded, and some of the staff from the X-ray Department helped to swell the throng. We were greeted with a very warm welcome, and plates piled with sandwiches and other Christmas fare were thrust into our hands, along with an invitation to help ourselves to a drink. I sat on the floor in the corner of the room and realised how tired I was. It was a strange way to be celebrating Christmas, at five thirty in the morning, I thought, but on consideration, most of the night staff would be sleeping throughout Christmas Day, and would be on duty again that night.

It was much later when I managed to make my excuses and make my way back to the reception desk to collect my coat. Dave was exchanging some heated words with a new arrival.

'I know you have had your bleeding piles for the last three months, but why wait until six o'clock on Christmas Day to do something about it? I'll book you in to see the doctor. You should have gone to see your own GP.'

'I could bleed to death waiting for him to turn out ...'

The singer had changed, but the song was the same.

I picked up my coat, waved to Dave and made for the door. Outside, the cold morning air was like wine after the stifling heat of the Department. I made my way to my car and began scraping the ice from the windscreen, when suddenly across the road the figures of three men came into view as they passed through a pool of light from the nearby lamp standard. One of the men was being supported by the other two, and they were dragging him towards the Accident and Emergency Department. They were all obviously very drunk. One turned his head and saw me.

'A Merry Christmas!' he yelled from across the street.

'And a Merry Christmas to you,' I replied.

I got in my car and headed for home.

Chapter 16

New Year's Eve

"Ring out wild bells to the wild sky,
The flying cloud, the frosty light:
The year is dying in the night.
Ring out wild bells, and let him die."

Thus wrote Alfred Lord Tennyson.

Perhaps in his day and age the advent of the New Year saw the rebirth of new hopes, and a new era of peace in the war-torn Europe of that period. But even peace can bring its problems.

New Year's Eve in Casualty was also wild, and the only bells ringing were the telephone bells. This night seemed to be the final extension of Christmas festivities and the ultimate stage of the celebrations. There was a tide of booze flowing as the fete reached its grand climax, and the drunks started arriving quite early, some anticipating the arrival of the New Year by twelve hours, and mingling with the normal flow of patients. My arrival on the scene was also earlier than usual, as I knew from previous experience that the department would be busy.

As I put on my white coat, Tracey the staff nurse beckoned to me and I moved over to her.

'What do you want, Staff?'

'You can help me solve one of life's greatest mysteries.'

'Eh?'

'A puzzle that's haunted mankind since the dawn of creation ...'

'Bloody hell!'

'... Our names will be emblazoned in all the scientific journals of the world.'

'Have you been hitting the bottle?'

'No.'

'Then what are you on about?'

'There's an inebriated Scotsman in the cubicles suffering from a head injury who needs undressing. Will you give me a hand? Then together we will discover the truth.'

'The truth?'

'Yes ... what a Scotsman wears beneath his kilt.'

'Are you joking?'

'No, and if you hear any rude noises it's from his bagpipes that are on the tray beneath the trolley.'

Angus McPherson was too drunk to bother about us as we attempted to undress him. He was both tall and broad in girth, and we had great difficulty in lifting him. He was arrayed in full Highland dress, and his kilt was stained from either drink or vomit.

After I had removed his shoes, Tracey bent down to remove his socks.

'Mind his dirk,' I said.

She stopped suddenly. 'His what?'

'His dirk. It's tucked in his sock.'

'My God, he must be deformed.'

'It's his dagger.'

'His dagger. Oh, I see what you mean. That's a funny place to keep it. Alright, I'll leave that end to you. How do I get his whitewash brush off?'

'You mean his sporran.'

'Well, it looks like one.'

Considering we had never undressed a patient adorned in complete Highland regalia before, we managed fairly well between us. True, there were problems with his kilt as we unwound what seemed several yards of material, with Tracey estimating how many skirts she could make out of it, and we were puzzled at first by his top half. But we did solve the mystery of what he wore under his kilt.

Unfortunately the code of ethics that exists at the hospital to safeguard the patients' interests prevents me from revealing what we discovered. However, Tracey was satisfied with what she saw. I can simply mention that he shopped at Marks and Spencers.

* * *

There are three types of drunk, according to my classification: the happy drunk, full of good spirits, particularly the sort that come out of a bottle. Singing and joking, they want to share their happiness with everyone around them, and also other things like being sick over you if you didn't take care. Then there are the sad drunks who want to tell you how their wives (or husbands) don't understand them, or speak about their dear departed mothers with nostalgic tears running down their faces. Finally, there are the fighting drunks who want to do battle with the whole world and usually end up fighting some poor innocent nurse in the Casualty Department.

Fortunately on New Year's Eve, most of the patients were of the happy variety. They were not always easy to deal with, but at least that extra degree of violence was absent, even from some of our well known patients, whom the staff treated with respect. It was unlikely that they had made any New Year's resolutions to be good, but rather they had been influenced by the general bonhomie.

Very often, the relatives or friends accompanying those seeking treatment caused more trouble than the patients themselves. Leading up to midnight, I was helping Alf the reception clerk to book in the new arrivals. The waiting room was already overflowing, the casualty officers were dealing with some seriously injured victims from a road accident, so the patients with minor injuries were kept waiting for treatment.

As I stood writing in the admission book, Alf gave me a nudge in the ribs.

'Bloody hell, Walter, we're being invaded.'

I looked up from my book and saw a host of women pouring through the doors. They were all in fancy dress, and their ages ranged from early twenties to late forties. They surrounded the reception desk and pushed people out of the way without any apology to get to the front of the queue. There was a general clamour of voices raised in protest, all yelling at once. A large, well-made woman wearing what looked like a German officer's uniform, complete with a swastika armband and carrying a whip in her right hand, shouted to everyone to be quiet, and she took command of the situation.

'Good God, Alf, we've got Hitler back,' I whispered.

Alf looked at her through the vent in the glass screen.

'Can I help you?' he enquired.

'Get a doctor to see my wife at once.' This wasn't a request, it was an order.

'What's happened to her?'

'We were having a party and she had a fall and banged her head.'

'Was she knocked out?'

'No.'

'I'll book her in. What's her name?'

'That's her, Little Bo Peep,' said Hitler, pointing with her whip to a young girl wearing a long flowered dress and a bonnet.

'Are you all her sheep?' asked Alf.

'Don't get funny with me,' said Hitler, waving her whip. 'You get a doctor at once.'

It took some time to establish that Bo Peep's real name

was Morgan, and that her marital status was single, although Hitler kept insisting that she was the girl's husband, and that the rest of the group would verify the fact.

'You'll have to wait your turn,' said Alf. 'You can see how busy we are, but I'll get a staff nurse to come and see the patient.'

'Nurse?' said Hitler. 'You get a bloody doctor at once, can't you see how the girl's suffering?' She started waving her whip about again.

The suffering girl concerned was now drinking a cup of coffee from the machine, and appeared to be sharing a joke with Minnie Mouse.

'I'll get the triage nurse to come and look at her, Alf, or we're likely to end up in a concentration camp,' I said.

Hitler's companions had now taken over the waiting room. Bo Peep and Minnie Mouse were now hugging and kissing, Maid Marion and Little Boy Blue, or rather Little Girl Blue, were locked in each other's arms, while a female Robin Hood watched with interest. Danny the porter viewed the group through the glass screen from behind the desk.

'Bloody lot of leslies,' he said. 'They've been in here before.'

'Leslies?' I queried.

'Lesbians. They have a party now and again and when they do, they go berserk. We had to get the police in last year to clear them out.' He wandered away shaking his head.

It was some time before the triage staff nurse came to see Bo Peep's head. She was quite a pretty girl, and to her embarrassment her entrance aroused several wolf whistles from the gay fraternity in the waiting room, causing her to blush. In spite of the threat of Hitler's whip, she told Bo Peep that her injury did not require priority treatment, and then promptly took refuge behind the reception desk.

‘A lot of men have made advances to me during my nursing career,’ she said. ‘But that’s the first time I’ve been propositioned by a member of my own sex.’

When at last Bo Peep’s name was called to see the doctor, the whole tribe flocked forward and followed her to the treatment area. Alf and I waited for Sister’s reaction, and it wasn’t long in coming. Supported by three porters, and led by Danny, the women were all driven back to the waiting room. Hitler’s voice could be heard above the din.

‘Let me stay with her, she’s my wife.’

Followed by Sister’s voice.

‘... If you don’t stop waving that bloody whip about, I’ll stick it up your arse ...’

* * *

Most of the staff regarded illnesses or injuries caused through drinking as being self inflicted, though this type of patient received the same attention as the rest. But on occasions like Christmas and New Year’s Eve, the drunks dominated the scene, causing a backlog for the staff and an extension of the waiting time for the genuine patients. As the minutes ticked away the over-crowded waiting room resounded with the sound of human voices. A radio playing pop music was somewhere in the dense crowd, and in one corner people were handing round bottles, while others were singing. Two of the porters were trying to appeal to those waiting to be quiet and have a little respect for the rest, but it had no effect. It was only with the arrival of the police, bringing in an injured suspect, that some order was restored. Most of the people in the waiting room were the friends or relatives of people waiting for treatment, and they were responsible for the uproar.

In the city centre it was traditional for the crowds to gather round the Clock Tower and in the Town Hall Square at midnight to greet the New Year. This should have been a happy occasion, but very often it was a cue for violence from a small majority of revellers, and many fights resulted. These affairs spilled over to other areas, and shop windows were broken and cars damaged.

Mr. Hung Lo, who owned a Chinese restaurant and take-away, was upset when his window was kicked in by one hooligan. The youth responsible for the incident had a badly cut hand and the police arrested him and brought him to the hospital for treatment. This was perhaps lucky for the offender, for when Mr. Hung Lo discovered where the man was, he decided that he would also like a word or two with him and made his way to the Casualty Department.

New Year's Eve should be a time of new beginnings, of forgiveness and joy, but alas there was no forgiveness or joy on the face of Mr. Hung Lo as he entered the waiting room, for he carried a large cleaver in his right hand which he waved about above his head. The crowd parted just as the Red Sea did for Moses, and there was a deadly hush as the singing and shouting suddenly stopped. Alf saw him approaching, and for once even he looked uncertain of what to do.

'I don't like the look of him,' he said. 'When I was young I used to read books about a chap called Fu Manchu. This must be his brother.'

He stood back from the desk in case the cleaver was going to be used to smash the screen.

'What's your problem, Sir?' he asked.

I don't know what Mr. Hung Lo's answer was, as his use of the English language was limited, but his intentions were quite clear when he started to swing the cleaver round his head like a shot putter.

'Get the Police, Walter, for God's sake.' Alf shouted to me. 'He'll chop my balls off with that thing.'

Being New Year's Eve, the two policemen were already in the department. One was in charge of the youth responsible for the window smashing, and the other was dealing with a drunk who was causing trouble. I dashed up to them.

'There's a Chinese man in the waiting room waving his chopper about. Can you come at once?' They must have thought I was drunk.

'Waving his chopper?'

'His hatchet ... his cleaver. I think he wants to kill someone.'

'Oh, I see what you mean. We can't have that can we now?' said the taller of the two, and they both made their way to the waiting room, with me following. All the patients and their friends and relatives now lined the walls, out of reach of the Hatchet Man who stood in the centre of the room waving his weapon, and yelling in some strange tongue.

The tall policeman recognised him immediately.

'Now Mr. Hung Lo, we don't want any trouble from you, just hand me that weapon. It's our turn now to go into the take-away business, and I'm starting with the hatchet.'

The other constable, coming from behind, grabbed Mr. Hung Lo's arm, and there was a volley of words from the restaurant owner. But then he relaxed his grip on the hatchet's handle, and allowed the policeman to take it away.

'Let's have you now,' said the tall constable. 'You had better come with us. You can't go round the city with an offensive weapon threatening people, even if some of the citizens deserve to be put on your menu. The one you are looking for would be a bit tough.' And with that he escorted Mr. Hung Lo from the waiting room.

There was an audible sigh of relief at the departure of Mr. Hung Lo, and a rush to the reception desk by the patients still waiting to be booked in.

Alf turned to me.

'A happy New Year, Walter.'

I looked at the clock. It was now well past midnight. On nights like this it was easy to lose track of the time.

'A happy New Year to you, Alf. I'm glad your wife's wedding present is still intact.'

I turned to the next patient. 'Can I help you, Sir?'

* * *

'Can you book a patient into St. Peter's Ward for me, Walter, when you're free?' Sister enquired. 'She's not conscious, and we don't know who she is. She has obviously been drinking and must have had a fall and cut her head. You'll find her with the staff nurse. The police will be along later to interview her.'

I discovered the patient in the corridor with the other patients, along with the nurse who was acting as escort to the ward. The girl lay on a trolley with her eyes closed, and in spite of the alcohol on her breath, I could also smell her perfume lingering in the air. She was a very pretty girl with short blonde hair, and her use of make-up added to her charms – red lips and discreet eye shadow.

I turned to the nurse. 'Nothing is known about her, then?'
'No, she was found lying in the street so someone called an ambulance.'

I duly filled out the admission form: Name and address unknown. I also put a line through the spaces that wanted to know her next of kin, her age, her religion and the name of her G.P., and handed the form to the nurse.

'Can you come with me to the ward, Walter, I'll need a lift to get her into bed.'

Although I was badly needed on the desk I could hardly

refuse such a request, and so we made our way through the queue in the corridor to St. Peter's Ward. The ward nurse on duty indicated the bed for the patient, we pushed the trolley alongside, and she unrolled the blanket that the patient was wrapped in.

'She's wearing some exotic undies,' the nurse said. 'It would cost me a week's salary to buy some like that.'

I caught a glimpse in the dim light of the ward of a red silken bra trimmed with lace. Her briefs were of a matching colour with the same trimming, and her red tights completed the colour scheme. I picked up the rest of the clothes from the tray beneath the trolley. Her coat, shoes and dress were also bright red, and I placed them on the locker at the side of the bed.

'A happy New Year,' I said to the nurse on the ward.

'The same to you,' she replied. 'You can make me happy by not bringing any more pissed-up patients here tonight.'

After waiting for the lift and wending our way through the silent corridors, it was about ten minutes before we finally arrived back at the Casualty Department. The scene hadn't changed and it seemed to be more chaotic than ever. One of the porters grabbed the empty trolley and dashed away with it, and I rejoined Alf at the reception desk. He looked up as I entered.

'Have you seen Sister? She's looking for you.'

'No. What does she want?'

'You'll find out.'

I pushed my way through the crowded area and found her.

'Did you want me, Sister?'

She looked up from the treatment card she was checking.

'Yes. You know that patient you have just taken to St. Peter's Ward?'

‘Yes, what about her?’

‘She’s not a her, she’s a him.’

‘Are you joking? It can’t be, she’s a female. I helped lift her into bed. She was wearing red undies. I saw them.’

‘Well, when they removed them, she appears to have developed a penis and two testicles, so you had better go back and remove her – I mean him – to a male ward. The staff will tell you which one.

When I returned to the ward the mystery man, who was still in a drunken stupor, was now attired in a cotton nightdress supplied by the hospital. He still had traces of make-up on his face, and his perfume still lingered in the air. He still looked pretty and feminine.

‘We’ve had to put him in that nightdress,’ said the nurse. ‘We don’t stock men’s pyjamas on this ward. His dress and undies are in the bag on the locker.’

I paused.

‘If the male patients see him like this, they’ll think it’s going to be a happy New Year.

* * *

As the time passed the crowd in the waiting room thinned slightly, but the situation did not improve, owing to the arrival of two badly injured patients from a road traffic accident and a cardiac arrest, both incidents needing the full attention of the doctors on duty. Alf was absorbing most of the abuse from the people waiting to see a doctor, and he remained very cool and polite considering the pressure he was under. It was only when a pushy young man tried to jump the queue waiting for treatment that he got rather heated.

‘I have Mr. Peter Piper outside in my car. Can you send a doctor to have a look at him?’ The young man said.

Alf looked at me, and I shrugged my shoulders.

'What's wrong with him?' asked Alf.

'He's hurt his arm.'

'He can't walk?'

'Of course he can walk.'

'Well you tell him to walk inside this building and I'll book him in to see a doctor. But he's got a long wait. If you look round you can see for yourself how many people are waiting.'

'But it's Peter Piper the television star. I'm his manager.'

Alf turned to me and in a loud whisper asked, 'Who's he when he's about?'

'He's on Top of the Pops. Don't you ever watch it?'

He turned to the manager. 'You'll have to ask him to come in, Sir.'

'I can't bring him in here among this crowd, they'll recognise him immediately. I don't want him mobbed. You send a doctor to see him. Peter Piper's a star and he's been hosting a local show.

'I don't care if he's Peter Pan, he's still got to be booked in,' said Alf.

It was now dawn and another year had been born. The remaining patients in the waiting room were slumped in their chairs. No longer were their voices raised in song, and the new year for most of them would still bring the same routine of work, the same worries as before, and perhaps the problems of an uncertain future. The hands of the clock moving past midnight on a certain day in a certain month cannot change our lives, only our hopes.

As I was getting ready to depart for home, the new-found peace in the department was shattered by the wail of bagpipes from the treatment area. Angus McPherson was now awake and greeting the New Year.

"Ring in the valiant man and free,
The larger heart, the kindlier hand;
Ring out the darkness of the land:-
Ring in the Christ that is to be."

Chapter 17

CHANGES

"The Moving Finger writes; and having writ,
Moves on; nor all thy Piety nor Wit
Shall lure it back to cancel half a Line,
Nor all thy Tears wash out a Word of it."

The hospital was like a living unit in the heart of the city, and as the city grew in size, so did the hospital. The long awaited extensions came to fruition, and phase two of the building work was completed in 1979. At midnight on Saturday, March 31st of that year, the Accident and Emergency Department officially moved to its new home.

When I arrived during the early evening, the reception staff had already started emptying the files and packing all the casualty cards in cardboard boxes, and the porters were engaged in moving the equipment that was unlikely to be required. It was the usual busy scene, and for the staff the work went on as normal, in spite of the impending move. Patients still had to be treated, phones answered, and it was just before midnight when I helped Michael the ambulance-man unload his last drunk to be treated in what was henceforth going to be called the "old" Casualty Department.

As the staff moved over after midnight, I stood alone in the eerie silence that surrounded me. The reception desk stood unmanned, the trolleys were all lined up in the corridor, and the curtains round the patients' cubicles were drawn back, revealing a black emptiness. I wandered along the passage and looked into the Fracture Room. White plaster still adhered to the single table, where so many Saturday sportsmen had lain while their injuries were treated. There was a deep sense of sadness as I stood thinking of all the people I had met in the department over the years. The silence of the waiting room was broken by the sound of my footsteps, and I wondered what my role would be in the new department. Would I be needed in the future?

When I joined the other staff in the new building the clock hands ticked over to April 1st, and I thought that moving on April Fool's Day must have some significance, but couldn't think what. Everywhere looked new and unused, and the whole area was just waiting for the incoming patients to give it the activity, the smells and noise associated with the old Casualty Department.

The new Resuscitation Room could now hold four patients instead of one, and there were cubicles for sixteen patients, apart from the side rooms. Further along the corridor was the Fracture Clinic, a much needed addition to the department, as well as a Gastric Lavage Room for stomach wash-outs, and a theatre for minor operations. The new Recovery Room and the Overnight Ward were also a great improvement on the old ones. The X-ray Department now consisted of five units, with a comfortable waiting area and dressing rooms. Luxury indeed! So I thought at the time, but I was to discover later that even the new department would soon prove to be inadequate with the passing years. Much later a separate Children's Facility was also added, and no longer were the young patients forced to share the main waiting room with the drunks and other adults.

There was a room behind the Casualty reception desk earmarked for the Porters' Lodge, but as the architects never consulted the staff about their working conditions, this was taken over to store the department records, much to the annoyance of the porters, who then went on strike. It was something of a dilemma for me. As they were my friends and I worked closely with them, I had no desire to be considered a strike-breaker, and so I did not go to the hospital for two weeks. As I drove to work every morning past the gates, I waved to the picket outside, who returned my gesture with a friendly thumbs-up sign. It was a sad sight, as this section of the staff was just as essential to the smooth running of the hospital as the other employees, yet they were always low on the priority list.

Their work was taken over by all sorts of people: medical students, clerical workers and general labourers, but fortunately the strike waned, and conditions returned to normal without the porters gaining any real concessions, apart from an admission that they did have an important part to play in the development of the hospital.

Working conditions slowly changed, the patient intake increased dramatically as the months passed, and it was necessary to increase the Casualty reception staff, as the single male clerk on the night shift could no longer cope on his own. It was during this period that I could divide my own working conditions into B.C. and A.C., meaning Before Computers and After Computers. It was then that the computer age caught up with the hospital. Not everyone could cope with the change. Ron, one of the night clerks, struggled for a time and soon retired, and although I was familiar with the system, I did not have the authority to access the program, and so my help in the reception area was limited.

Hospital security was always a problem. As the new extensions came into use, from 1979 onwards, the porters were replaced by the hospital's own security staff. It was surprising the items that were stolen. Pictures would disappear from the walls, furniture would go missing, purses were taken off the wards, and at night offices and administrative areas were raided.

Even an E.C.G. monitor went missing. The hospital car park had the reputation of losing more cars by theft than anywhere else in the city; this was apart from the large number of vehicles that were damaged in the course of theft. Video security cameras were installed to sweep the vital areas of the hospital, but the vastness of the buildings that were always open to the public made it a thieves' haven, and a security officer's nightmare.

The extensions continued, the hospital spread its tentacles to meet the demands of the city it served, and in line with government policy at that time it opted to become a Hospital Trust. With the new policies and changing methods, the staff were apprehensive about job security due to the Trust's desire to save money. Some domestic duties and the shops that were run by voluntary labour were contracted out to private firms, and the kitchens adopted the freeze-and-cook style of catering. Some nurses were put on short term contracts, and no one seemed very happy with the changes. Even the portering services were scrutinised and reviewed to try and save money. Yet the administrative staff at the centre of power seemed to grow out of all proportion to the rest of the hospital workers, and they had strange titles to describe their roles.

The introduction of new medical procedures produced re-engineering teams, whereby selected members of the nursing and medical staff could carry out comprehensive tests on patients in minutes rather than hours, although the term 're-engineering' built up a picture in most people's minds of doctors and surgeons standing around waiting for their victims with spanners and screwdrivers in their hands. New jargon was also used to disguise old methods, and members of staff were somewhat cynical about the changes.

The pressure on the Accident and Emergency Department increased as the years passed, and it was estimated that four out of every ten patients who were booked in for treatment could have been treated by their own G.Ps. There was a great demand for beds through the Central Bed Bureau that served the local hospitals, and during the busy periods it was not uncommon for some patients to be left lying on their trolleys for several hours before they could be allocated one. This particularly affected the elderly, and caused them great distress. With an increase in our ageing population, it was questionable whether the planners were aware of the impending crisis.

In two and a half centuries the hospital had grown from a small unit set in the fields beyond the city's walls to a huge complex that was still pushing its boundaries outward, and swallowing up streets and buildings that stood in the way. With the advent of new techniques in medical science, and the public demand for better hospitals, there will always be constant changes taking place, but let us hope that they will be for the better.

Epilogue

When I depart, let there be no sad songs,
No crystal tear to cloud the amber eye,
No sighs, no regrets.
But rather pluck a jewel from your treasure chest
of memories,
Hold it to your breast, and wish that I was there.

It was time for me to go. I hate goodbyes. Memories of long lingering farewells and tears shed at railway stations and airports came flooding back, and the talk of swift reunions that would never take place. Now there would be no one to cry at my departure, nor would my name be emblazoned in the hall of fame. I was like a shadow passing by, leaving no mark. But the hospital remained. It had doubled in size since I had first started there. The once over-crowded casualty department where the doctors, nurses, porters and radiographers mingled together and shared the laughter, the tears and the violence, was now gone. It had given way to a new building, splintered into separate departments for the different groups.

New faces brought new methods and procedures that were strange to the staff, and with the growth of the hospital came the growth of the administration, but not the communication. The waiting room with its modern furnishings, complete with the large television set to pacify the waiting patients, no longer housed the ghosts of Helen and her bottles of Guinness, or Steptoe the blanket stealer. Paddy Murphy was found wrapped in newspapers on a park bench, deep in his last sleep. His humble obituary commanded six lines in the local press. Numerous faces without names passed before my eyes. Wherever they were now, it was time for me to join them in that ever rolling stream called time.

I passed the reception desk on my way out; the computer had started to print the daily records. The micro-chip revolution had reduced the patients' names to numbers. Alf the reception clerk waved to me as I went through the door. It was four o'clock on a Sunday morning, the first bright light was showing over the hospital's tower blocks. I moved over to my car that was parked in front of the entrance and glanced back.

Yes, it was right that I should depart. I was part of the past, the future now lay with the others.

Goodbye Casualty, may you never lose the warmth and compassion towards the people you serve.

The pox doctor's clerk got into his car and drove away without looking back.